"*The Whole-Body Workbook for Cancer* provides an update of progress in natural treatments for cancer along with practical guidelines for health, which are therapeutic in their own right and are the 'work' of this book. Thus, Dan Kenner's book replaces the helplessness and fear of cancer with useful information and positive action to improve the results of cancer treatment overall and promote a better quality of life. Positive action requires work; this book points you in the right direction. Now the work is up to you."

—Richard A. Kunin, MD, president of the Society for Orthomolecular Health
Medicine and author of *Mega-Nutrition*

"*The Whole-Body Workbook for Cancer* is a timely and important addition to the growing number of books addressing the critical importance of diet, exercise, and lifestyle in the cancer survivor. This book can provide a map to both better health and wellness for patients. Only in the last several years has research proven that improved survival as well as quality of life is possible when a healthy diet and lifestyle are adopted by cancer patients. Whether patients are in treatment or well on the road to cure, this important book will promote the healing that is open to all patients."

—Donald Boyd, MD, internist, oncologist, and curriculum director for
Complementary and Alternative Medicine and Nutrition at Yale Medical School

"I fully endorse *The Whole-Body Workbook for Cancer* written by Dan Kenner; this is a comprehensive and well-written workbook."

—Mark Rosenberg, MD, founder and director of the Institute for Healthy Aging in
Delray Beach, FL

"Dan Kenner provides an excellent journey into the world of healing from the most feared illness of our era: cancer. He is authoritative, yet empowering to the reader. A most important work for patients, family, professionals, and students of healing."

—EnRico A. Melson, MD, MPH, FACPM, DAAPM, ABIHM, MHT, KSJ, cofounder of the Integral Medicine Institute in Beverly Hills, CA

"*The Whole Body Workbook for Cancer* offers the information and steps you can take to not only survive, but also to stay strong and support your body while receiving cancer-fighting treatments. Based on research, this book provides the tools to improve your diet, manage your emotions, and lift your spirits so you can get through this challenging time. And these are the same tools that can help you remain healthy in your life beyond cancer, as a survivor."

—Judith McKay, RN, OCN

# THE
# WHOLE-BODY
# WORKBOOK FOR
# CANCER

## A COMPLETE INTEGRATIVE PROGRAM FOR INCREASING IMMUNITY AND REBUILDING HEALTH

DAN KENNER, PH.D., L.AC.

NEW HARBINGER PUBLICATIONS, INC.

## Publisher's Note

*This publication is designed to provide accurate and authoritative information in regard to the subject matter covered. It is sold with the understanding that the publisher is not engaged in rendering psychological, financial, legal, or other professional services. If expert assistance or counseling is needed, the services of a competent professional should be sought.*

Distributed in Canada by Raincoast Books

Copyright 2009 Dan Kenner
New Harbinger Publications, Inc.
5674 Shattuck Avenue
Oakland, CA 94609
www.newharbinger.com

Acquired by Jess O'Brien; Cover design by Amy Shoup;
Edited by Nelda Street; Text design by Tracy Marie Carlson

Library of Congress Cataloging-in-Publication Data on file with the publisher

Kenner, Dan, 1950-
  The whole-body workbook for cancer : a complete integrative program for increasing immunity and rebuilding health / Dan Kenner ; foreword by EnRico Melson.
      p. cm.
  Includes bibliographical references.
  ISBN-13: 978-1-57224-674-4 (pbk. : alk. paper)
  ISBN-10: 1-57224-674-X (pbk. : alk. paper)  1. Cancer--Alternative treatment.  I. Title.
  RC271.A62K46 2009
  616.99'406--dc22
                        2009038432

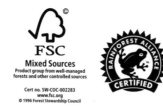

11   10   09

10   9   8   7   6   5   4   3   2   1            First printing

This book is dedicated to my clients and patients, past and present, from whom I've learned, in so many ways, what life is really about.

# Contents

# Foreword

A disastrous medical diagnosis is a transforming event. It's natural to experience great fear when you feel there is a threat to your life. Quite likely you have felt confused about what to believe, conflicted about *whom* to believe, and unsure how to proceed. This chaos can lead to a crisis of trust, including trust in your own intuition. In this situation, many people find themselves feeling hopeless, and hopelessness is the epitome of disempowerment.

In order to not succumb to your natural fear or feelings of powerlessness, you need the love and support of friends and family. You need confidence in your professional team of health care providers, and you need information that will help you feel empowered to make the decisions that best suit your needs and inclinations. Perhaps the shock of a cancer diagnosis has led you inward to a deeper level of self-awareness. After this soul-searching, you need the type of information and structure that gives you a sense of power and the ability to make choices that foster optimism and hope.

We human beings don't know all of the factors that shape our destiny, but we do have the capacity to make decisions that have a vital impact on our physical and spiritual quality of life. While it is unfortunate that environmental factors have contributed to an increase in the incidence of many cancers, we also have witnessed a considerable improvement in the overall survivability of cancer and improvement in quality of life for many people living with cancer. No one invokes cancer or looks forward to receiving such a diagnosis, but you can certainly learn many powerful and useful means of integrating mind, body, and spirit, strengthening your innate responses to coping positively with such challenges. At the very least, one need not approach cancer with the sense of helplessness that so often accompanied the diagnosis in prior years.

I believe that true healing is the experience of alignment among the physical, emotional, mental, and spiritual aspects of our being. This understanding has been a part of spiritual and healing traditions throughout the world and throughout history. In this book, Dan Kenner draws on his scholarship, his expertise, and his compassionate care to offer a spectrum of options and resources to address all of the factors that influence well-being and healing. A truly comprehensive approach such as this one can optimize cancer treatment, improve quality of life, and perhaps even extend longevity. Whether you have cancer yourself or are helping a family member or friend through it, the approach laid out in this book will offer you both hope and practical tools.

I wish you the best on your journey.

—EnRico Melson, MD, MPH, FACPM, ABIHM, ABAARM, KSJ
Integral Medicine Institute
Beverly Hills, California
June 2009

# Acknowledgments

This workbook wouldn't have been possible without support from my wife, Corinne, and son, Daniel; thank you for your patience and encouragement. I am also grateful to several researchers and health care practitioners, whose dedication inspires me and whose sharing of experience and willingness to engage in dialogue have been a source of great value: Michael Broffman, OMD; Nancy Carroll, L.Ac.; Robert Felt; Helmut Keller, MD; Jean-Claude Lapraz, MD; Michael Lipelt, DDS, ND; Michael McCulloch, Ph.D.; Buxiang Sun, MD; and Dale White, L.Ac. The editorial support and advice of the staff of New Harbinger Publications has been a key element in organizing and structuring the contents of this book.

# Introduction

Nothing short of being a victim of armed robbery induces a feeling of powerlessness as effectively as a cancer diagnosis. The combination of anger, grief, and fear over what to do can be disabling. The central purpose of this book is to help you overcome the feeling of powerlessness and to give you the necessary tools to empower yourself. Feeling powerless can be as hazardous to your health as any environmental toxin or damaged gene. This is a key point because there are many reasons to feel powerless when you or someone you love is faced with cancer. First and foremost, you might feel powerless facing the fact that cancer is considered an incurable disease. If modern medical science can't cure it, what can laypeople do? Turning our care and chances for survival over to medical professionals, often in large medical institutions, is humbling, especially since medical personnel sometimes make decisions for our care without our full participation.

Powerlessness has even been the subject of scientific investigation. A study at the University of Pennsylvania showed that the immune systems of test animals with tumors rejected the tumors at a slower rate when the animals were powerless to escape stressful stimuli. The results demonstrated that the feeling of powerlessness accelerates a tumor's progression (Visintainer, Volpicelli, and Seligman 1982). Self-empowerment not only makes you *feel* stronger but is also necessary for survival.

We also get the message from scientific reports in the media that the new medical frontier is genetic technology, which conveys, inadvertently perhaps, that the cause of disease is in our genetic inheritance and that medical technology is learning how to correct this built-in defect. Genetic markers for various types of cancer and other diseases have been widely reported (Petrakis and King 1976). We wait anxiously for progress to catch up to the modern health scourges, while what we can do for ourselves is often de-emphasized or devalued. If cancer is caused by some kind of inborn defect, what can we possibly do about that?

The fact is that we can do a lot, and what we do can help decide the outcome of our longevity and well-being, and the success or failure of our treatment. The role of genes may predispose you to certain types of health problems, but genetic defects directly cause only a very small percentage of diseases (Human Genome Project Information 2008). The news that's not so widely reported is the well-documented evidence that a toxic environment and modern dietary habits are the real causes of cancer and its dramatic upsurge over the last sixty years (King, Marks, and Mandell 2003). I find relief and empowerment in this type of information. Instead of waiting for a technological breakthrough or a miraculous cure, you *can* do something about your health, both in prevention and treatment—right now.

# DIET AND LIFESTYLE MATTER

Research conducted over the last few years has gradually led to new thinking about cancer. This book outlines strategies on using nutritional and lifestyle changes to help you reduce any tendencies in your body to develop cancer. Chapter 1 explains that there's a new age in cancer treatment dawning that's based on new scientific understanding of what promotes cancer and allows it to take hold, and even seize control, of the body's normal defense mechanisms. Dr. Dean Ornish's pioneering human clinical research in 2005 gives us evidence that how we conduct our lifestyles, from diet to stress management, makes a difference. He has shown that a whole lifestyle conversion—including diet change, specific supplementation, exercise, and stress reduction methods such as yoga, breathing, and visualization—can affect the development of cancer. Dr. Ornish studied ninety-three men at an early stage of prostate cancer who were diagnosed by biopsy (Ornish et al. 2005). The group choosing the lifestyle program didn't use any type of conventional cancer therapy, while the control group had no treatment at all. Both groups were monitored by regular PSA (prostate-specific antigen) blood tests. Ornish was aware of previous studies showing that foods such as tomatoes and soy products seemed to reduce the risk of prostate cancer (Snowdon, Phillips, and Choi 1984) and that some foods, such as certain dairy products, eggs, and meat, can increase it (Allen et al. 2004). This was the clinical trial that showed that the progression of prostate cancer can be stopped, or even reversed, by changing diet and lifestyle alone.

At the end of a year, the results were published. They showed that six patients, all from the control group, had dropped out, because MRIs or other diagnostic tests of cancer activity showed that their tumors were growing at a rate that made it necessary to look at other options, such as surgery, chemotherapy, or radiation. None of the members of the group undergoing diet and lifestyle change showed any negative developments. The PSA (prostate-specific antigen) markers had actually decreased in this group. The results showed a very significant difference between the two groups (Ornish et al. 2005).

Many of us have an urge to become more actively involved in our health care rather than be merely passive about it. According to the *Journal of Clinical Oncology*, 60 to 80 percent of cancer patients now combine complementary treatment with conventional treatment. The article encourages the oncology community to be willing to communicate openly, adopting a nonjudgmental communication style, and research the possible interactions among drugs, herbs, and vitamins (Richardson et al. 2000).

The oncology community is oriented toward heroic treatment methods: chemotherapy, surgery, and radiation. There are no chapters on diet or lifestyle in the textbooks of this medical specialty, despite the fact that mainstream medical research has known about the key role of diet in the cause and progression of cancer since the 1970s (Carroll and Khor 1975). Since that time, an abundant and convincing body of scientific evidence has accumulated, not only diet research but research on the effects of stress, trauma, and environmental conditions on the immune system and the incidence of cancer. Taken as a whole, this scientific research gives us a rational foundation for designing a personal strategy.

Many of the books on cancer survival, especially books on alternative medicine, focus on diet and supplements. There's an ongoing hope for a "cure," a nontoxic cure, if possible. However, there's much more to improving health or fighting disease than finding a cure. It's simplistic to think of any one thing as a possible cure. "Does it work?" is the wrong question to ask about a new supplement or drug. I believe that many methods being promoted as a cure have helped someone. The real questions are "What works for whom and why?" and "What works for me?" Creating new habits is the core strategy of any type of change. Sometimes what you take out of your life is more important than what new remedy or medication you put in.

There's probably no treatment method, conventional or otherwise, that's a stand-alone treatment. Success of any therapy depends on the inner resources of your body and mind. Cultivating and reinforcing these inner resources is the key to success. Some people have robust vital resources, some have robust spiritual resources and strong willpower, and some are deficient in inner resources and have fragile health. Regardless of the starting point, it's almost always possible to create some type of improvement in the status of your health and well-being. Your focus doesn't necessarily have to be on conquering disease. I suggest adopting the goals of longevity and quality of life. This book explains how to become knowledgeable about and skillful in natural health care to achieve longevity and a higher quality of life.

# CHOOSE YOUR TEAM AND YOUR APPROACH

The most important advice for how to use this book is that if you have cancer, or any major health challenge, don't to try to do it all alone. Carefully choose a team of professionals and try to weave them into a support net for your healing process. A complementary health care provider—whether a medical doctor, osteopath, chiropractor, naturopath, or acupuncturist—can play an important role on your team. The stereotype of an untrained quack exploiting desperate, gullible late-stage patients is much less common than imagined. Work with your loved ones too.

Share with them what you learn, or let them do the research and share it with you. If you're alone, find a support group to avoid the stress of trying to go it alone.

Because so much information is available on diet, lifestyle, and natural therapies, it's necessary to sort through it all carefully. In this book I emphasize methods that science has soundly established and that will benefit the largest number of readers. It's important to understand the scientific literature on diet, supplements, lifestyle, and stress. There are also methods, foods, and supplements for which the scientific literature is sparse or nonexistent. Chapter 1 presents the scientific principles supporting this book's recommendations. This background knowledge is very important. Even if the terminology is unfamiliar at first, the ideas will soon be familiar.

Despite the ongoing barrage of optimistic claims from leading cancer research institutions that new breakthroughs are around the corner, a growing number of researchers and patient advocates are discouraged by the lack of progress. For most cancers, if a tumor has metastasized, the chances of survival haven't improved since the "War on Cancer" was declared in 1971. What *has* changed is the new focus on natural medicine and complementary health care. Most of the improvement in longevity of cancer patients is the result of improvements in diet and lifestyle, and early detection (Leaf 2004).

Cancer's widespread occurrence suggests that many people haven't had access to the kind of information provided in this book. The promotion of lifestyle improvements has become more conspicuous in the last few years but is still the subject of controversy. An ample body of research evidence now supports the use of various nutrients, herbs, and supplements to slow down the progression of the disease and extend life span (Block et al. 2007). Some supplements have even been specifically developed to support conventional cancer therapy to protect the immune system from the ravages of chemotherapy and radiation treatment.

A bewildering volume of information is available on how to treat cancer with unconventional methods. Some of these methods or remedies are supported by scientific data, and others have only been tested informally or not at all. Most people desire to combine "the best of both worlds," by using conventional medicine and attempting to integrate it with complementary approaches. In most cases conventional treatment *can* be integrated with alternative treatments. Certain diet and lifestyle measures greatly increase your odds of benefiting from conventional treatment. Using certain supplements can also enhance the likelihood of success. The question is, and always will be, what's best for you?

People who are serious about their survival and quality of life adopt a positive approach to their health challenges. Resources and discoveries abound that can help you use positive thinking to its full advantage, not only to improve your quality of life but also to create better physical health in tangible and measurable ways.

Whether you're a cancer patient, a cancer survivor, or the loved one of either, this book is designed to help you find a personal pathway through the ocean of information now available in print and online. The book covers the most important things that every person affected by cancer needs to know about diet, supplements, stress reduction, immune-system support, detoxification, exercise, and dealing with fear and the residual effects of old traumas. It covers basic information on some of the most common types of cancer, and reviews both conventional and emerging treatment methods. I'm optimistic about the scientific breakthroughs that are on the horizon.

# TAKE CONTROL OF YOUR EXPERIENCE

Research from the Netherlands (van Baalen, de Vries, and Gondrie 1987) has shown that "spontaneous remission" of cancer occurs much more frequently than the previously estimated 1 in 60,000 to 100,000 cases (Cole 1981). I've certainly observed this in my own experience with people who choose to take control of their life experience. I've even observed cases in which people rejected conventional therapy completely and had successful results, although I'm not recommending that you do this. Statistics primarily keep track of those patients who are in the medical system and who undergo conventional therapy. Spontaneous remission is considered to be nothing short of a miracle and is sometimes attributed to divine intervention. I certainly won't dispute the possibility of divine intervention, but perhaps divine intervention "helps those who help themselves." Perhaps we can develop a "technology of miracles" so that we can create our own miracles. As you explore this book, I hope that this technology of miracles will strike you as common sense.

# CHAPTER 1

# Understanding Cancer

Cancer is uncontrolled, unlimited cell growth. It's completely chaotic, creating a structure that has no function other than its own expansion. Unlike the division of normal and healthy cells, which occurs in a regulated and systematic fashion that maintains the body's tissues, cancer cells ignore signals in the body that limit further division and growth. Cancer cells also lack a property that normal cells have, which is to self-destruct after dividing a certain number of times. This programmed cell death is called *apoptosis*. Cancer cells continue to grow unabated and expand in their local environment, and can also spread to other parts of the body, which is called *metastasis*. It would be incorrect to say that researchers understand all the causes and mechanisms of cancer. But even though there are still many mysteries to be uncovered, a lot is known about some of the mechanisms that promote cancer and about the relationships among lifestyle, radiation, chemical exposure, and other causes. Numerous theories provide useful models for the basis of treatment.

We're actually entering an era in which there's a new scientific understanding of cancer. We all know about the devastating effects of chemotherapy and radiation, such as nausea and vomiting, hair loss, fatigue, anemia, and loss of immunity. The new understanding of cancer is leading to treatments that combat the underlying mechanism of the disease, rather than just destroy the tumor and hope the immune system will recover. While we may not yet have a new generation of medical treatments, you can take advantage of what's known in this "new paradigm" and apply it to your lifestyle and treatment plan.

We may think of cancer as a gross abnormality, a glitch in the body's normal pattern of functioning, but in reality we all carry cancer "seeds" inside of us. All living organisms manufacture defective cells, which are the source of cancerous growth. Several internal mechanisms prevent this abnormal growth from getting out of hand in most people. If any of these mechanisms fails, it can lead to an upsurge in the number of abnormal cells. Such mechanisms are the means of surveillance, detection, and destruction of these deviant cells as they form. Failure or impairment of the body's normal methods of detecting and dismantling renegade cells can result in a health condition that's both dangerous and difficult to correct. But equally important is the fact that if these microscopic cancerous "seeds" we all produce fall on fertile soil, they'll grow into a menace. The internal environment of our tissues and fluids, and their metabolism make fertile soil for cancer "seeds" to develop under certain specific conditions.

There are four conditions that promote cancer development and growth:

> Oxidative stress

> Inflammation

> Blood vessel formation (*angiogenesis*)

> Lack of immune system competence or surveillance

Consequently, there are four ways presently known to inhibit the development and growth of cancer:

> Reduce oxidative stress

> Create conditions that discourage inflammation

> Prevent formation of new blood vessels

> Restore immune competence or surveillance

In this chapter we'll take a look at each of these.

# OXIDATIVE STRESS

Dr. Otto Warburg (1883 to 1970) won the Nobel Prize in Physiology or Medicine in 1931 for his discovery that cancer cells function in a state of oxygen deprivation and replace normal oxygen respiration by fermenting sugar into lactic acid. In other words, cancer cells depend on sugar, because they have abnormal oxygen metabolism. Although this observation has not led to treatment methods, diagnostic PET (positron-emission tomography) scans are used to detect cancer because they measure the parts of the body that consume the most glucose (blood sugar). This observation has also led to the hypothesis that we should avoid sugar in the diet because it's fuel for cancer (Warburg 1966), since sharp rises in glucose cause sharp increases in insulin and IGF (insulin-like growth factor), both of which stimulate growth and inflammation. Hypoxic cancer cells use the sugar in a fermentation process that prevents them from regaining normal oxygen utilization. PET scans monitor tumor development by tracking glucose metabolism.

Oxygen is necessary for the health of our cells. We can't live more than a few minutes without it. But at the cellular level, too much oxygen results in toxicity by creating *reactive oxygen species* (*ROS*) like "free radicals," whereas too little oxygen impairs normal cell function (*hypoxia*). Maintaining oxygen within normal levels is important throughout life, but it's critical when there's rapid cellular development, whether it's normal or abnormal. Too much reactive oxygen in the cells, called *oxidative stress*, is a potential cause of cancer and other diseases (Toyokuni et al. 1995), but too little oxygen in tumor cells correlates with acceleration of the development of malignant cells (Höckel et al. 1993). Furthermore, low tissue oxygenation may also be a contributing factor in metastasis (Brizel et al. 1996). Oxidative stress damages membranes, proteins, and DNA. It causes aging and degenerative diseases when the body loses its capacity to neutralize and detoxify the ROS by-products or to repair the damage they cause (Fiers et al. 1999). The body's cells have an "antioxidant" defense system. Oxidative stress is imposed on cells partially from a decrease in antioxidant protection or a failure to repair oxidative damage.

Vegetables and fruits are antioxidants, along with most unsaturated vegetable oils, teas, and many herbs and spices. Cooked foods, especially cooked and smoked meats, tend to be more oxidative. Tobacco smoking is a particularly strong source of potentially stressful oxidants. Making sure that the diet includes many vegetables and fruits is one way to support our natural cellular antioxidant system. Vitamins, trace minerals, and amino acids are also antioxidants, along with many other substances used as supplements for their antioxidant effects. Whether or not cancer patients should continue taking antioxidant supplements during radiation treatment in cancer therapy is a confusing issue today because of wide media coverage of a flawed study (Bairati et al. 2005) indicating that taking antioxidants could reduce survival time in patients undergoing radiation therapy.

The ten-year study concluded that two synthetic antioxidant supplements had a harmful effect on cancer patients receiving radiation therapy. This was the first placebo-controlled, double-blind, randomized trial assessing the effect of supplementation with antioxidant vitamins during radiation therapy. The researchers, Dr. Bairati and colleagues, claimed that the recurrence rate of cancer was 40 percent higher among the patients receiving the antioxidants (Bairati et al. 2005). The media picked up this report and sounded the alarm to use caution about taking antioxidants until new evidence could be provided by future trials.

In December 2007, Dr. Bairati and her Quebec colleagues published an update of their previous study. They had discovered that the group at risk from taking the synthetic antioxidants was limited to the subpopulation of cigarette smokers, people who had continued smoking during radiation treatment (Meyer et al. 2008).

Antioxidants are not a panacea and certainly aren't a stand-alone treatment for cancer, but they play a vital and fundamental role in a successful outcome. Recent studies have shown that combining chemotherapy with antioxidants can reduce 57 to 70 percent of the adverse effects of chemotherapy and improve quality of life (Nicolson 2005), and that some antioxidants actually increase the effectiveness of chemotherapy (Chinery et al. 1997).

# INFLAMMATION

Another condition that promotes and supports cancer is inflammation. Inflammation is sometimes depicted in popular scientific articles as a disease, and anti-inflammatory drugs are often used to treat diseases like arthritis and asthma, but inflammation is actually a healing process. The immune system uses enzymes to break down damaged or morbid tissues, which creates the typical symptoms of heat, pain, redness, and swelling. The immune system is signaled by *blood platelets*, the blood cells that gather together to form blood clots. Platelets release a substance called *platelet-derived growth factor* (*PDGF*). This alerts the white blood cells of the immune system, which produce numerous substances that serve as chemical messengers, setting the tissue-repair process in motion.

At the first stage of inflammation, the blood vessels in the neighboring tissues dilate, thus opening the pathways from the white blood cells to the wounded area. Next the lesion is sealed off as the platelets start the process of blood clotting. The chemical messengers open the surrounding tissues, making them porous so that the tissues can be saturated with immune cells to control infection. Finally, they activate cell multiplication and the construction of blood vessels to bring oxygen and nutrients to the new cells that are forming. This is the normal process of tissue repair when there's injury to any part of the body. New cell growth stops when the new tissues are in place. The white blood cells stop the inflammation process and go back to surveillance mode.

These same processes can go out of control, however, and be used to subvert the body's health and integrity. An inflammatory process that doesn't completely resolve can not only become a source of ongoing discomfort but also prepare a fertile place for cancer "seeds" to grow. The idea that cancer is a "wound that does not heal" goes back to the 1800s, when one of the fathers of modern pathology, Rudolf Virchow, observed that cancers often appeared in parts of the body that had been injured, sometimes repeatedly (Dvorak 1986). Over a hundred years later, an article called tumors "wounds that do not heal," reviving this concept (ibid.). Chronic inflammation from an irritation, such as tobacco smoking, can lead to lung cancer, or irritation from asbestos exposure can lead to mesothelioma. *Colitis*, inflammation of the large intestine, is implicated in some cases of colon cancer. Infections, such as *Helicobacter pylori*, the stomach ulcer bacterium found in stomach cancer, can also be the source of inflammation. In some viral infections, viral genes can have an effect on cell transformation. Hepatitis B and C viruses are implicated in liver cancer. HPV (*human papillomavirus*) is a viral infection implicated in cervical cancer.

Cancer takes the healing process of inflammation and subverts it for the nourishment of cancerous growth. Just as immune cells are activated to repair lesions, cancerous cells must produce inflammation to sustain their growth and proliferation. They manufacture large quantities of the same substance chemical messengers use in the healing process (cytokines, prostaglandins, and leukotrienes). These substances promote cell multiplication and make the surrounding barriers porous and permeable, enabling the cancer cells to infiltrate neighboring tissues and circulate through the blood and lymph systems to form distant colonies, the process known as metastasis. After normal tissue healing, the production of these substances ceases, but cancerous growth drives a large quantity of these "pro-inflammatory" chemicals to the perimeter of the adjacent tissues to *stop* apoptosis, the genetically programmed cell death used by the body to promote normal cell turnover and prevent chaotic cell growth. Cancer cells, protected from this process of cellular death, are thus able to grow unchecked. And the more the tumor grows, the more pro-inflammatory chemical signals it secretes to fuel its growth.

In this way, inflammation can be both a cause of cancer as a precondition and an effect of cancer, because tumors accelerate the inflammatory process in a vicious cycle. Premalignant tumors are wound-like in nature. In the early stages of development, the body treats tumors as wounds. During later tumor growth, the tumors themselves drive the inflammatory process.

## Two Key Chemical Messengers Involved in the Inflammation Process

There are two key inflammatory chemical messengers found in most inflammatory processes. The first is a cytokine called *interleukin-6* (*IL-6*). *Cytokines* are chemical messengers that carry information in the immune system, the most famous of which is *interferon*, but there are dozens of cytokines. IL-6, a cytokine that appears to be especially important in the inflammatory process, is a sophisticated biosensor for environmental stress, reacting to even minor challenges to the equilibrium of the cellular environment.

Control of IL-6 may depend on the second key inflammatory chemical messenger, a protein complex called *nuclear factor kappa B* (*NF-kB*). NF-kB is a protein complex that's a transcription factor (a protein that transfers information to DNA). NF-kB is involved in how cells respond to stimuli such as stress, cytokines, free radicals from oxidative stress, ultraviolet irradiation, bacteria, and viruses. NF-kB is associated with various cytokines besides IL-6 that mediate the inflammation process. Researchers at University of California, San Diego, believe that NF-kB may be the most fundamental target of all for cancer therapy. Blocking its production makes cancer cells vulnerable to treatment and prevents metastasis (Karin and Greten 2005). Blocking NF-kB can also cause tumor cells to stop proliferating, to die, or to become more sensitive to the action of antitumor agents. Almost all anticancer agents are NF-kB inhibitors, according to Albert Baldwin of the University of North Carolina (Marx 2004), and the new holy grail of cancer research is to find ways to inhibit this factor (Karin et al. 2002). Fortunately there are many natural substances that can accomplish this, including those found in herbs (Leclercq et al. 2004), green tea (Wallace 2002), fruits, and fatty acids (Packer, Kraemer, and Rimbach 2001).

## Inflammation and Stress

When the stress-response system and immune system are activated during inflammation, they interact through the hypothalamus, which is the brain's master control center for adaptation, and the adrenal glands. The fight-or-flight response is caused by the release of *adrenaline*, which makes us more alert and focused, and by *cortisol*, which converts protein to energy and releases our stored sugar. The adrenal response rapidly increases our heart and respiratory rates, and blood pressure while releasing energy, tensing our muscles, and slowing digestion. When the stress is chronic, the body doesn't return to normal and stays in an aroused state. High cortisol levels can cause agitation, fatigue, depression, and poor memory. The fight-or-flight type of stress response, when the heart rate increases, the breath becomes deeper and more rapid, and the muscles tighten, is also associated with reduced NF cell activity and higher IL-6, the pro-inflammatory cytokine. This results in the development of inflammatory syndromes, such as rheumatoid arthritis, and behavioral syndromes, such as depression. Thus, some diseases may be caused by both inflammatory and emotional disturbances (Sternberg et al. 1992). A study at Emory University School of Medicine found that men diagnosed with depression had significantly higher levels of IL-6, the pro-inflammatory cytokine, and NF-*k*B activity, showing a link between emotion and inflammatory diseases (Pace et al. 2006).

# BLOOD VESSEL FORMATION (ANGIOGENESIS)

Cutting off the nutrient supply of a tumor or any other pathological growth sounds like a logical idea, but when it was first proposed, it was so revolutionary that it was met first with skepticism. Dr. Judah Folkman (1933 to 2008), a surgeon working in a U.S. Navy laboratory, came up with this idea in 1961 while researching the use of freeze-dried hemoglobin in place of fresh blood on long tours of duty at sea (Folkman et al. 1971). He tested the hemoglobin to see if it could sustain thyroid glands extracted from a rabbit. As a side experiment, he implanted cancer cells from mice into the gland and then irrigated the gland with the artificial blood. Tumors developed, but their growth stopped at a certain point. Something obviously prohibited them from growing any further. When he reimplanted the same cancer cells back into a live mouse, however, the tumor grew rapidly, almost without restraint. The contrast was dramatic. Dr. Folkman noticed by looking through a microscope that the difference was that the rabbit thyroid lacked a complex of tiny blood vessels.

Dr. Folkman spent the rest of his career establishing his theory that malignant tumors could not grow larger than the head of a pin without blood vessels supplying nutrition, which became known as the *angiogenesis* (*angio*, "blood vessel," plus *genesis*, "creation") *theory*. He also believed that the tumor must secrete some substance that stimulates this new growth of blood vessels, an *angiogenin*. He speculated that if there was a way to block this new creation of blood vessels, an *angiostatin*, the growth of tumors could be stopped, which would be an entirely new way to treat cancer.

Skepticism of Folkman's theory dissipated over the next two decades. The discovery of angiogenesis factors (ibid.) and angiostatins created the foundation for a whole new area of cancer research and treatment. The next step was to see if angiostatin could really prevent or stop the cancerous tumor development. Michael O'Reilly, an associate of Dr. Folkman, induced cancer in twenty mice with a virulent type of transplantable cancer cell known for its ability to metastasize rapidly. After implanting the cells, he injected the angiostatin protein into half of the mice and then let the disease take its course with both groups. The group without any intervention presented the expected ravaged lung tissue from the metastatic cancer cells. The angiostatin-treated group, however, developed normal, pink tissue, apparently free of disease (O'Reilly et al. 1994).

Angiostatin not only prevented cancer from forming, but also, in experimental models, it was able to reduce existing tumors to a minute size without damaging any normal structures, even blood vessels. Normal blood vessels are a stable part of the infrastructure of all tissues, and their growth is self-limiting. But cancer-tumor blood vessels, like cancer cells themselves, are fragile and have chaotic growth. The possibility of a nontoxic cancer therapy is revolutionary in conventional cancer treatment.

Drugs with the properties of angiostatin have since been developed, and there are several foods and natural remedies with angiostatin-like properties (see chapters 5 and 6).

# LACK OF IMMUNE SYSTEM COMPETENCE OR SURVEILLANCE

Does such a thing exist as immunity to cancer? Dr. Zheng Cui, an associate professor at Wake Forest University, discovered a mouse that seemed to be *immune* to cancer. Although not originally a cancer researcher, Dr. Cui (Cui et al. 2003b) often injected a virulent type of cancer cells (sarcoma 180, known as "S-180 cells") into mice to induce the formation of antibodies for use in his experiments. The mice seldom lived longer than a month. Usually 200,000 S-180 cells are enough to induce cancer, but one mouse survived—even after a second try. There was no formation of cancer or abdominal swelling in this mouse. Dr. Cui repeated the procedure with 20 million S-180 cells and then 200 million of the toxic S-180 cells, but there was still no change! It seemed that this mouse had a trait completely unexpected and unimagined: natural immunity to cancer. This trait was genetically transmissible, because the second generation of offspring of this mouse, dubbed "Mighty Mouse," inherited this mysterious cancer resistance. The mice were able to survive a dose as high as 2 billion S-180 cells, enough to comprise 10 percent of their body weight. This is the equivalent of transplanting an extremely malignant fifteen-pound tumor into a human adult.

One generation of mice was used in a cancer experiment after an interval of several months. To Dr. Cui's surprise, these mice quickly developed tumors and swelling. With disappointment, he realized he would be unable to carry out any further experiments on this miraculous immunity phenomenon. Perhaps it had been only a strange scientific anomaly. The next surprise, however, was that the mice recovered to perfect health after simply being left alone. The explanation that emerged was that the strength of the inherited immunity diminished with age.

Accounts of spontaneous regression of advanced-stage cancers have appeared in the medical literature for decades, but no scientific model existed to explain how this could happen. Here, for the first time, was an experimental model of spontaneous regression of cancer with test animals in controlled and observable laboratory conditions. The mechanism that appeared to give these mice immunity to cancer was very high activity of a certain type of protective white blood cell. The S-180 cells were attacked by white cells that attached themselves to the invading cells, punctured them, and destroyed them. This type of white blood cell is called a *natural killer*, or *NK, cell* (Hogan and Basten 1988).

NK cells are often called the "sentinel" cells of the immune system. They provide the first line of defense against pathogens, such as bacteria and viruses, but also abnormal cells, such as cancerous or virus-infected cells. NK cells are a type of large white cell that's filled with granules. NK cells target tumor cells, other abnormal cells, and a wide variety of infectious microbes but leave normal cells alone. Unlike some white blood cells, NK cells don't need to recognize a specific antigen before attacking and destroying a target cell, which is why they're called "natural" killer cells. Unlike other white cells, they don't engulf and ingest target cells but, rather, attach to them and inject chemicals that erode the membranes of the target cells until they burst. In many chronic and degenerative diseases, including AIDS, the activity of NK cells is measured to indicate how long a patient will live.

## NK Cells and Stress

Numerous studies have shown that reduced NK cell activity correlates strongly with stress. In many cases, NK cell activity is the only immune system factor that can definitely be related to the psychological damage of trauma or chronic stress. A trauma can also suppress immunity for long periods. People with a history of *post-traumatic stress disorder (PTSD)* have shown significantly weakened immune competence even years after the initial trauma (Kawamura, Kim, and Asukai 2001).

A variety of stressors that can suppress NK cell activity have been researched: physical injury caused by accidents, surgery and medical treatments, nutritional deficiencies, emotional trauma, grief, hormone imbalances, and many others. Reduced NK cell activity occurs so consistently from trauma or chronic stress that it can be considered a marker in blood tests for stress-related disorders. So, NK cell activity is a very important measurable link between mind and body in medicine. Even self-criticism can decrease NK cell activity (Strauman, Lemieux, and Coe 1993).

Not only is NK cell activity an important link in mind-body medicine, but other evidence also shows that it's a factor—maybe a key factor—in chronic disease (Whiteside and Herberman 1990). The breakdown of the scavenging function of NK cells and other white cells may be the origin not only of cancer but also diseases such as hepatitis, diabetes, chronic and opportunistic infections, and even autoimmune diseases (Hogan and Basten 1988).

Even if the immune system is unable to completely destroy all cancer cells, recent research shows that it can at least hold them at bay and maintain long-term stability. Scientists at the Cancer Research Institute (CRI) in New York, in collaboration with researchers at five other academic institutions, have shown (Koebel et al. 2007) that dormant cancer cells are kept in a dormant state by the immune system. This dormant, or "equilibrium," state has been observed previously. Autopsies have often shown tumors that never developed into cancer. Cancers that were *latent* in an organ donor have become *active* in organ recipients. Organ recipients have to take immune-system-suppressing drugs to prevent rejection of the transplanted organ. Of course, this can create conditions where the latent cancer can grow. These scientists hope to find ways to use the immune system to contain existing and potential cancerous growth. They also hope to become able to explain how some tumors seem to suddenly stop growing and go into a lasting period of dormancy.

The four conditions known to promote the development of cancer—oxidative stress, inflammation, angiogenesis, and lack of immune system competence or surveillance—are not independent factors but are very much interrelated. As you'll learn in chapter 3, each of these four factors can be modified through our own efforts. We can maintain a high-antioxidant diet and use antioxidant supplements. We can control inflammation with diet and lifestyle, and use supplements that prevent development of unwanted new blood vessels. Stress affects the balance of behavioral, cardiovascular, and immune system activity, but we can use supplements to address our stress issues, thereby boosting the function of the immune system.

# CHAPTER 2

# Diagnosis and Treatment Notes

Though I've always been oriented toward complementary treatment methods, I remain supportive of conventional science and technology. In fact, I believe that there are serious scientific breakthroughs coming in the near future that will transform cancer diagnosis and treatment. I don't foresee anything that would change the basic recommendations in this book to strengthen body, mind, and emotional resilience, but I do think we'll see safer, more effective therapies and improved quality of life for cancer patients and their loved ones.

## EXCITING NEW BREAKTHROUGHS

The breakthroughs that are on the horizon could be the subject of an entire book. Gene therapies that can make cancer cells self-destruct and keep them from affecting normal cells have been tested successfully in animal studies (Xie et al. 2007). Nanotechnology is producing tiny nanoparticles that can absorb infrared light and heat up malignant tumors to destroy them but leave healthy tissues undamaged (O'Neal et al. 2004).

The theory that cancer may grow from stem cells may shed light on why most cancer therapies have been unsuccessful. If the daughter cells of the stem cells are destroyed, but not the stem cells themselves, new malignant cells will continue to be produced (Cho et al. 2008). This theory also opens the door to new therapies that could someday target the stem cells and clear out cancer at its root. Early cancer of the esophagus can be treated with Cryospray, which freezes the abnormal cells, causing them to slough off and allow healthy tissue to grow in their place. Another cancer-killing device, a cancer *filter*, can capture cancer cells from the blood. This device, developed at the University of Rochester Department of Biomedical Engineering, could be used to take out cancer cells and prevent metastasis, but it also appears to collect stem cells, which could be used for a variety of therapeutic purposes.

Used for years in Europe, hyperthermia has recently started to make headway here in the United States. It's well known that cancer cells are more sensitive to heat than normal cells and can't survive a high temperature (Armour et al. 1993). Clinical trials at the University of Texas may result in FDA approval for this method (Bull 1982; Bull et al. 1979), which is practically considered to be a mainstream treatment in some parts of Europe (Nielsen, Horsman, and Overgaard 2001).

# CHANGE IS IMMINENT

In the past, too many conventionally trained doctors ignored diet and lifestyle as important factors in patient care, but this is rapidly changing. Today we see the beginnings of a movement toward *integrative medicine*, combining diet, lifestyle, and alternative treatment approaches with conventional care. This is even happening in the cancer community at such well-established institutes of learning as the University of Texas and UCLA. The conventional methods of treatment, surgery, chemotherapy, and radiation focus entirely on getting rid of tumors. In many cases the cancer is considered a local disease, and treatment chases after it if it spreads. The new paradigm, as emphasized by the World Cancer Research Fund's "Expert Report" of November 2007 (www.wcrf.org/research/expert_report/index.php), is that lifestyle factors such as nutrition and exercise are not only useful for prevention but also a necessary part of treatment.

The internal metabolic condition of the whole body is where the cancer "seeds" we all produce are planted. If the "soil" is fertile for cancer development, it'll grow. The body's internal environment, as well as the fluid that bathes every cell of our bodies, is actually referred to as the "terrain" in some schools of thought in European medicine. In late nineteenth-century France, Louis Pasteur and the great physiologist Claude Bernard debated whether the "germ" or the "terrain" were more important. Pasteur eventually agreed with Bernard that for infections, treating the terrain, or the internal environment, was more important than just killing the germs (Simon 2006).

By using the strategies in this book, we can restore our metabolism, our internal cellular environment, to keep cancer seeds from growing. This approach creates an integration of medicine and healing that will optimize the outcome of any necessary medical procedures.

# METASTASIS: THE BLIND SPOT OF CANCER RESEARCH

What really matters in cancer treatment is stopping metastasis, because it's what's responsible for death in the great majority of cancer patients. Research on metastasis, however, makes up less than half of 1 percent of funded research studies (Moss 2004). One of the mysteries of metastasis is that at least 30 percent of metastases appear in locations that are distant from, and often not even linked by a blood supply to, the primary tumor (Demicheli et al. 2008). Another mystery is how one type of cancer cell may spread rapidly, while another spreads very slowly or not at all. This can be related to the idea of cancer cells as "seeds." If the conditions in the body are fertile for these cancer "seeds," which are tiny clusters of cancer cells, also called *occult cancer cells*, they'll take hold and spread. If not, they'll die out or be destroyed. Research is under way to see if substances called *monoclonal antibodies* can inhibit metastasis (Brooks et al. 1993). Given the danger of metastasis, it's important to look at the whole picture of the body's condition: immunity, toxic exposure and burden, and levels of oxidative stress and inflammation. This is where lifestyle truly makes a difference.

# CANCER SCREENING AND DIAGNOSIS

Screening and diagnosis both use medical procedures and diagnostic devices, but there's an important difference. Screening procedures are used to check the condition of people who are symptom free. Ideally the purpose of screening is to detect a problem at an early stage so that it can be treated sooner in the hope of a better outcome. Diagnosis is the use of medical procedures to determine the cause of a suspicious symptom or sign. While there's no infallible screening method for detecting the early stages of cancer, there are important considerations for each type of method in use.

## Breast Cancer

**The Benefits of Self-Examination:** Two large studies from Russia and China (Kösters and Gøtzsche 2003) analyzed data of over 388,000 women and found that death rates from breast cancer were the same among women who rigorously self-examined their breasts and those who didn't. There were almost twice as many biopsy operations in the self-examination group. Despite these grim facts, it's still important to learn what's normal and to feel the breasts regularly for signs of any change. Look for new lumps or hard spots in the breast or armpit, any dimpling or puckering of the tissue, drawing inward of the nipple, or any swelling or change in the size of your breast. Look for asymmetry between the left and right breasts, as well as redness, nipple discharge, and tenderness or pain. Report any changes at all to your health care provider.

**Mammograms:** Mammograms continue to arouse controversy even among responsible medical authorities. A Danish study published in the *Lancet* several years ago concluded that widespread mammogram screening is unjustified and that research showing a benefit from it was flawed (Olsen and Gøtzsche 2001). That may not be the last word, but the radiation hazard of repeated mammograms must be considered, since radiation is a well-established cause of cancer. The effects of the radiation hazard of mammograms accumulate over your lifetime. The usefulness of mammograms is also limited when the breast tissue is dense, such as when a woman is nursing or taking hormone replacement therapy. According to the National Cancer Institute (2007), mammograms miss up to 20 percent of breast cancers. Mammograms find tumors only once they've reached a certain size, but changes in physiology can occur before tumors actually form. The breast, thyroid, and lung are particularly sensitive to radiation (Curtis et al. 2006). Some people have genetic sensitivities to radiation. David Goldgar, former chief of the Genetic Epidemiology Group at the International Agency for Research on Cancer (IARC) in Lyon, France, suggests that women who are "members of families known to have BRCA1 or BRCA2 mutations may wish to consider alternatives to X-ray, such as MRI" (Andrieu et al. 2006). Mutations of the BRCA genes predispose women to breast or ovarian cancer. In considering risk versus benefit, the accuracy issue is significant. The cumulative risk of false positives in women at age 50 after five screening mammograms is 24 percent. After ten screenings, it's 47 percent. For women between ages 40 and 49, the risk is 30 percent after five screenings and 56 percent after ten screenings (Elmore et al. 1998). Breast thermography and MRIs are two other options that can give an enhanced perspective.

**Thermography:** This diagnostic method can detect the possibility of breast cancer much earlier, because it can form an image of the early stages of angiogenesis. Thermography uses a camera that detects heat, and while it isn't as accurate as mammography for detecting slow-growing tumors or those that don't have increased blood vessel formation, it can show a tendency toward tumor development before detection is possible by any other means. It's also extremely safe for the breast tissue because it introduces no radiation of any kind. However, since it's a new procedure, there are fewer experienced practitioners, and women who've undergone thermography have been told not to worry when there actually was cause for concern. False and missed diagnoses are a pitfall of all of the screening techniques.

**MRI:** The MRI is also a very safe diagnostic procedure, and it will detect most of the tumors missed by mammograms. The weakness of MRI is its inability to distinguish a benign mass from a malignant one. Despite this downside, high-risk patients may wish to avoid exposure to the radiation used in mammograms in favor of an MRI. For women already diagnosed with breast cancer, the MRI can be a useful follow-up tool for planning surgery and evaluating the result. Studies have shown that a presurgical MRI can significantly affect the treatment plan (Orel and Schnall 2001). If you choose to have a breast MRI, be sure to choose a medical center that uses breast MRI coils and that's staffed with radiologists who are experienced in reading and interpreting the images.

I recommend using more than one method of evaluation. If you wish to limit your radiation exposure and want to overcome the limitations of solely using the mammogram, consider using either MRI or thermography in combination with the mammogram. I believe that mammograms have significant flaws and that the radiation exposure should be minimized, but both MRIs and thermography lack national standards for breast imaging, whereas national standards for mammography have been in place for years.

## Prostate Cancer

The PSA test is the test traditionally used for prostate cancer screening. Its limitations are well known; it's a marker for inflammation but not specifically for cancer. Very high PSA levels or sudden surges in the PSA level in a short period, however, *can* be a reliable indicator. A urine test recently developed for prostate cancer detection, the PCA3 assay, promises to be a more accurate and specific diagnostic tool. The urine test screens for four different RNA molecules and was accurate 80 percent of the time in early trials of prostate cancer testing (Marks et al. 2007).

## Colon Cancer

Over 145,000 Americans are diagnosed with colon cancer every year, and more than 50,000 die from it (Jemal et al. 2006). If you go for a colonoscopy, be aware that cancers are more likely to be missed if the colonoscopy is performed in an office setting. It's also essential to have the procedure done by a specialist. Colonoscopies done as an office procedure, rather than in a hospital, actually tripled the risk of missed colorectal cancers in men and doubled the risk in women (Shah et al. 2007). Another important factor is that most family physicians and internists are trained to look for polyps, but flat lesions, also called *flat adenomas*, which don't protrude as much as polyps, are five times as likely to be malignant as polyps (Zauber, O'Brien, and Winawer 2002). Nonspecialists are 77 percent more likely than gastroenterologists to miss the cancer in men, and 85 percent more likely to miss it in women (Bressler et al. 2007). Most nonspecialists are not as likely to be aware of the importance of these flat lesions.

A typical sign of colon cancer is rectal bleeding or blood in your stool. Look for changes in your bowel habits for more than a couple of weeks. Look for diarrhea or constipation (bowel movements three times a week or less). Blood in the stool that comes from far up in the digestive tract isn't bright red but looks like coffee grounds. Also look out for persistent abdominal discomfort, such as cramps, gas, or pain; abdominal pain with bowel movements; weakness; fatigue; and unexplained weight loss.

Many people avoid the colonoscopy out of fear and resistance to the invasiveness of the procedure. One alternative to colonoscopy is the MRI, though it's not as reliable as colonoscopy. Another, newer alternative is *CT colonography*, also called *virtual colonoscopy*. The 3-D images obtained simulate what's seen in conventional colonoscopy. This new technique is 90 percent sensitive for polyps greater than 1 centimeter, and 50 percent sensitive for polyps with a 5 millimeter diameter (Mulhall, Veerappan, and Jackson 2005). A factor in the blood that may indicate colon cancer could necessitate a blood test to screen for it, which could help determine who's more at risk by not getting a colonoscopy (Cui et al. 2003a).

## Ovarian Cancer

The difficulty in treating ovarian cancer has always been the lack of early symptoms, which leads to late diagnosis. Ovarian cancer is the fourth leading cause of cancer death among women in Western countries. New research on breath analysis could lead to an early-warning diagnostic procedure. Touraj Solouki, a chemistry professor at the University of Maine, is working in conjunction with researchers at Pine Street Foundation in the San Francisco Bay Area. Solouki is using a large array of sophisticated electronic equipment to find a molecule indicating the presence of ovarian cancer. The researchers at Pine Street use dogs trained to identify a diagnostic scent. They've already demonstrated that the dogs can identify lung and breast cancer by smelling patients' breath with an accuracy rate of over 90 percent (McCulloch et al. 2006a). Breath samples that the dogs identify as positive for ovarian cancer are frozen and sent to Professor Solouki for analysis. If the key chemical can be identified, electronic Breathalyzers could be developed as diagnostic equipment. Researchers in Göteborg, Sweden, are also using dogs to diagnose and even distinguish different grades of malignancy. Their research so far indicates that early-stage and late-stage ovarian cancers have the same scent (Horvath et al. 2008).

## Lung Cancer

Early screening for lung cancer is almost nonexistent. Symptoms to look for include a persistent chronic cough, a feeling of being out of breath, chest and shoulder pain, coughing up blood, fatigue, and weight loss. CAT-scan screenings are used for high-risk patients to try to detect it earlier. There's a high rate of survival if surgery is performed at an early stage (Shah et al. 1996). Breathalyzers for early detection are in development and being tested with humans for early lung cancer detection.

# CONVENTIONAL CANCER TREATMENT

**Surgery:** Aggressive treatment to surgically remove malignant tumors is now being challenged by the idea that surgery can spread cancerous cells throughout the system. Researchers from Harvard University; University College, London; the University of South Carolina; and the National Tumor Institute, Italy, have published papers (Demicheli et al. 2008) showing that removal of a primary tumor could result in development of malignancy at distant locations. In other words, leaving cancerous tumors intact, rather than surgically removing them, may restrain the development of malignant cells in distant parts of the body, a finding that could lead to a new theory of metastasis and a rethinking of the aggressive strategy of removing malignant tumors as soon as possible.

*Radical prostatectomy* is the removal of a cancerous prostate gland. Andrew Vickers, a researcher at Memorial Sloan-Kettering Cancer Center, and his research team tracked the rate of recurrence of cancer following radical prostatectomy of 7,765 patients. According to Vickers, the rate of recurrence was directly related to the surgeon's experience. Patients operated on by a surgeon who had done the procedure only 10 times had a recurrence rate of 18 percent, compared to an 11 percent recurrence rate with surgeons who had performed the operation at least 250 times (Vickers et al. 2007).

A new tool for the surgeon is the robotic surgical system. Robotic prostatectomy is a less invasive method of prostate removal that results in a shorter hospital stay, less pain, lower risk of infection, less blood loss and scarring, and a faster recovery time. It enables the surgeon to perform the operation through tiny openings instead of a standard line incision. The surgeon directly controls every maneuver. Robotic prostatectomy has been used in thousands of prostate cancer procedures around the world.

A relatively new procedure, called *high-intensity focused ultrasound* (HIFU), presents an alternative to surgery. HIFU destroys cancerous tissue by heat rather than conventional surgery. The precision of HIFU allows the surgeon to accurately target the tissue to be destroyed without damaging surrounding tissues, thus reducing the overall trauma. HIFU is not yet available in the United States but is approved for use in Europe, Latin America, the Caribbean, China, and Japan. FDA clinical phase trials I and II have been performed in the United States, and plans are underway to start the final, phase III, FDA clinical trials (www.pcaresearch.com/about-the-study.html). Over 13,000 men have been treated with HIFU worldwide (Chinn 2005). If you want to consider this treatment, thoroughly discuss your case with your urologist to determine its appropriateness for you.

**Chemotherapy:** Drugs for cancer chemotherapy are the second largest category of drugs in the United States after cholesterol-lowering medications (Kolata and Pollack 2008). Because chemotherapy drugs don't selectively kill cancer cells, they're destructive to the bone marrow (where red and white blood cells are manufactured), the digestive tract, the hair follicles, and sometimes other systems, such as the heart and nervous system. Doctors are being urged to use caution in offering this harsh cancer treatment, especially to terminally ill patients, because chemotherapy often does more harm than good.

Critics of chemotherapy also point out that its rationale is to reduce the tumor, which isn't necessarily a factor in long-term survival. A drug is considered to be effective even if it only partially shrinks a tumor in tests. Chemotherapy has a high success rate in certain types of cancer, such as testicular cancer and Hodgkin's disease. It's always important to find out the success rate, not only for tumor reduction but also length of survival time, associated with any chemotherapy protocol prescribed for your condition.

A type of chemotherapy called *extreme drug resistance* (EDR) *testing* has been available for several years. It exposes tumor cells to chemotherapy drugs in a glass dish in the laboratory to determine if the cells are resistant to drugs. This testing isn't perfect and, like every innovation, is the subject of scientific controversy. The cancer cells and the drugs may interact differently in the body than in a laboratory setting, but this procedure may improve the selection process by eliminating drugs from consideration if the cells exhibit a pronounced resistance to them.

The use of a gene test called Onco*type DX* may help many women with breast cancer skip chemotherapy or choose lighter versions of it, while maintaining their chances of recovering from the illness. The test can determine whether or not a patient would benefit from chemotherapy by measuring the activity of twenty-one genes that can predict a woman's risk of recurrence. It's hoped that Oncotype DX will help doctors determine when to hold off on using chemotherapy or use it more selectively.

**Radiation:** Radiation has its risks and benefits. It can destroy rapidly dividing cells at the edges of tumors that surgery might miss, which could lead to a recurrence of the disease. It can eradicate cancer cells that don't respond to other forms of treatment. Radioactive seed implants can destroy cancer cells in a very localized area, sparing surrounding tissue (Wang 2000). Radiation can reduce the risk of breast-cancer recurrence, but one of the trade-offs is an increased risk of damage to the heart (Hooning et al. 2007). Some of the side effects of radiation include nausea, hair loss, fatigue, and low blood count, especially for white blood cells, although the bone marrow can also be affected. Patients also experience skin reddening and dryness, as well as drying up of mucous membranes of the digestive or respiratory tract, resulting in a variety of symptoms. Dryness of salivary glands can be a considerable source of discomfort, and scarring and thickening of connective tissue can occur over time. *Oral mucositis* (cells of the mouth rapidly dividing), loss of taste, difficulty swallowing, and erectile dysfunction are other side effects. Leukemia, multiple myeloma, secondary tumors, and thyroid disease can result, even years later, from high levels of radiation exposure (Wang 2000).

**Individualized Therapy:** Individualized therapy is one of the holy grails of medicine. One-size-fits-all, "disease-centered" treatment is only effective for certain patients, more or less by chance. In the case of cancer, as with any other disease, every person is different, even to the extent that each tumor is genetically different. With the stakes so high in cancer treatment and with frequent severe side effects from chemotherapy drugs, "targeted treatment" is gradually becoming available. Although imperfect, such treatments employ several tests and methods that can improve your odds of getting a more customized treatment. The idea of individualized therapy came to popular attention when the story of Dr. William Fair, a urologist at Memorial Sloan-Kettering Cancer Center, used a cancer vaccine specifically developed for him from his own colon cancer cells. Dr. Fair, previously skeptical of alternatives, used Chinese herbs to complement his treatment and grew to appreciate the benefits of a range of complementary approaches (Groopman 1998).

Many new innovations in cancer treatment are on the horizon. For the sake of both safety and thoroughness, women should explore alternative approaches to breast-cancer screening. New options are also becoming available for diagnosis of prostate, colon, and ovarian cancers. Finally, new testing methods are available that may help individualize cancer treatment.

# CHAPTER 3

# The Seven Elements That Build Health and Longevity

When you get a cancer diagnosis, you feel as if you have only one chance to make the right decisions. You need to make these decisions based on your best judgment and a thorough analysis of the most important factors. This book covers seven important elements that build health and longevity. Today a lot of information is available on options and strategies, and this book will only scratch the surface of possibilities. Collecting information is only part of the process. Feeling in your heart what's right for you is decisively important. Collecting information will help you with this process, but base your decisions on what you feel in your heart as well as your head. Whether or not we have a disease diagnosis, we all want life extension. However, I believe in pursuing the concept of life *expansion* as one of our healing objectives.

Establish your objectives, and be prepared to receive and record inner promptings. In chapter 10 you'll see how there's another "brain" besides the one in your head. Our inner promptings come from other sources of intelligence within us. Develop and discuss your plan with someone who knows you well, and stay open to possibilities. Your longevity and quality of life are worthy of your best effort.

**Element 1: Detoxification.** Detoxification is the process of internal cleansing. It goes right down to the cellular level and has many stages. Some extreme detoxification programs are successful. While I've seen people heal without using such extreme programs, some people feel that it's necessary.

**Element 2: Diet.** This is the opposite of "out with the bad." Maintaining a healthy diet is about bringing in nourishment and strength. It's an important issue today, because our modern diet has been an important cause of what are known as "diseases of civilization." There's almost no doubt that changes from more traditional diets have contributed to the cancer prevalence we see today.

**Element 3: Supplements.** Supplements are a part of our diet that provides concentrated nutrients or "functional foods" that help our bodies meet health challenges when ordinary foods aren't enough.

**Element 4: Lifestyle.** This encompasses how we interact with our environment. Are we savvy to some of the toxic or dangerous elements in our environment today? When radium was first discovered, it was touted as a medical miracle for everything from impotence to baldness. X-rays were a novelty that people exposed themselves to just to see the bones of their hands and feet. Today, we know the dangers of radiation. Our environment now has other dangers that aren't well known, but as with X-rays in the past, the information will spread, and we hope it won't be too late. On the positive side, it's important to enjoy the natural environment and get enough fresh air, sunlight, and exercise.

**Element 5: Exercise.** We all know about the importance of exercise, but it's especially important for cancer patients. Fatigue is often a symptom of cancer as well as a side effect of treatment. It may seem counterintuitive, but exercising, rather than resting quietly, is recommended for cancer-related fatigue (Sood and Moynihan 2005). Exercise increases efficiency of circulation, not just in the arms and legs but also the deep circulation in the abdomen, where your internal organs reside, which is important for overall health as well as for successful cancer treatment. Efficient circulation brings fresh oxygen and nutrients to the internal organs, and drains their waste products at a faster rate.

**Element 6: Emotional healing.** We need to understand, in a tangible way, the importance of emotional healing. This chapter contains strategies for healing old traumas, some of which you might not have heard of, but it's important food for thought.

**Element 7: Psychospiritual healing.** This goes more deeply into the realm of the intangible. You can take advantage of healing opportunities and methodologies regardless of whether or not you're a believer in a metaphysical world.

# BRINGING IT ALL TOGETHER

A breakthrough in any one of these elements of healing can affect everything else. A psychospiritual breakthrough can supersede everything else. On the other hand, good diet and exercise can help make you more likely to have an emotional or psychospiritual breakthrough. People used to fast to induce visions or to connect themselves with their intuitions or a higher power.

I don't recommend fasting, because I think that most of us aren't ready for it and that it could backfire. However, I do recommend "fasting with food," as you'll see in chapter 4.

Each of the next few chapters has information for you to consider and a questionnaire to fill out at the end. Some of the best advice I can give anyone is to look for your "blind spots." Even if you're an avid diet and natural-food enthusiast, you may carry around a lot of judgment and attitude, and be unwilling to look at your emotional life.

In my case, exercise is the blind spot. I have a good diet, take care of my emotional and spiritual well-being, and don't have a lot of toxic lifestyle habits. I'm an expert on supplements and natural medications, but exercise is a challenge for me. If I exercise, is it right for me? Do I benefit? Tremendously, even from a moderate amount. It's my blind spot. Even though I've tried to master all the other elements while keeping exercise in the background, exercise remains just as important for my health as for anyone else's. That blind spot holds special power, so watch for it. I've seen exercise enthusiasts whose diets consist of mostly junk food, containing lots of sugar. They're in such good aerobic condition that they feel no pain from this. But sooner or later, it catches up to them. Some people scoff at spiritual practices, psychotherapy, or emotional-release techniques. Be open to the idea that some real power may be available for you in something that you currently resist. People who meditate or are openly spiritual may seem "holier than thou," but there just might be something beneath the surface.

While the questionnaires at the end of chapters 4 through 10 aren't intended as a comprehensive lifestyle analysis, they're aimed at helping you clarify where to focus your attention. It's easy to plan your exercise program if you're a sports or diet fanatic, but if there's a missing link or you have a blind spot, the questions can help you identify important areas to focus on. It's my wish that all readers of this book develop all the personal power and freedom they can.

## FINDING YOUR BLIND SPOT

Do you have a blind spot? Write out a plan for how you'll focus your life-expansion strategy:

_____

_____

_____

_____

_____

_____

_____

# CHAPTER 4

# How to Detoxify

Most people think of detoxification in the context of drug abuse. "Detox" and "rehab" are interchangeable terms among the Hollywood jet set. In this case, *detoxification* means to optimize the body's ability to eliminate waste, that is, anything not needed as a nutrient. The main organs of elimination are the liver, the large intestine, and the skin. Many of us have experienced detoxification. The classic hangover is detoxification. The heroin addict quitting "cold turkey" feels extremely sick from detoxification. The jitters people get from quitting smoking or stopping a coffee habit are forms of detoxification. The important principle here is that when you're buzzed on alcohol, you're intoxicated, but when you're hungover, that's the healing. It's not a good feeling. A classic healing crisis—sometimes called a *Herxheimer reaction* or a *Jarisch-Herxheimer reaction*, and sometimes just a *Herx* for short—is a feeling of malaise. The symptoms are flu-like, sometimes accompanied by nausea, headache, fatigue, muscle tightness and pain, and migrating pains. Besides these symptoms, any chronic symptoms or health condition you've had could flare up.

## Levels of Detoxification

1. *Addiction:* Most people feel a lot better once they've let go of any dependency on coffee, sugar, or alcohol.

2. *Digestive tract:* Do you thoroughly digest your food? Do you have a bowel movement every day? Do you eliminate thoroughly?

3. *Fluid system:* Fluids from both the blood and lymph circulatory systems bathe the cells, providing nutrients and draining away metabolic waste products.

4.   *Tissues:* Detoxifying at the level of the tissues takes longer than the other levels—months and even years—because accumulated waste and congestion of the cellular environment has to be opened up and drained away through the fluid system or, as we'll see, the skin. The tissue level is where tumors reside.

# GENTLE DETOXIFICATION: THE FIVE-DAY DIET

Some cancer patients have gotten well by undergoing an intensive detoxification program, requiring the support of trained practitioners, family, and friends, but this is more work than most people are willing to do, and some of the detox programs demand that you avoid conventional treatment. However, this book encourages gentle detoxification that can complement conventional treatment, because most people I've consulted with prefer to combine conventional and complementary treatments. If you take prescription drugs, it's very important to discuss with your prescribing physician your plan to go on the detox diet before undertaking it.

While diet reform is important, your attitude toward it is even more so. Most people embark on diet reform with the attitude that they want to be "good." This approach is not about good or bad in the sense of giving up the "bad" things forever. There's definitely a place for discipline, but I believe in using it strategically and, at least in the beginning, in short bursts. This greatly expands the learning and adapting process. In the next chapter, on cancer-fighting foods, you'll learn that some foods have antioxidant, anti-inflammatory, immune-boosting, and other healthful characteristics. You can use this knowledge as guidelines to follow as you adjust to change.

This gentle detox approach is for a specific period, five days, in which you unburden your liver and digestive tract, giving them a rest while you eat nutritious, simple foods. What can we accomplish with this? We certainly won't change our health condition significantly in five days. What we *can* do is not only give the digestive organs a rest but also regain our health compass. After five days of this very simple diet, you'll become *sensitized*. And repeating this diet twice a month for three months will help you become very clear about what works for you and what doesn't. Most people don't experience any kind of healing-crisis reaction while on this type of diet.

If you hope to prevent a recurrence of cancer, a five-day diet period, twice a month, is enough. If you're actually facing a cancer challenge, make it your goal to lengthen the five-day period to around ten days at a time. Invariably you'll change the length of the period to suit your needs as you get used to the diet and learn more about what your body is telling you. What's your body telling you now? For many people, it's saying that it's time for a cup of coffee or perhaps a candy bar. Maybe it's telling them, "It's been a rough day, so it's time to have a drink." If this is you, don't worry about it. I'm not asking you to give up anything. In fact, I think it's very unhealthy to tell yourself that you can't have the things you love that are "bad" for you. All I'm asking for is five days at a time.

Let's consider coffee, sugar, and alcohol: These are not foods; they're drugs. A drug takes energy out of the system, whereas a food puts it in. To help you understand what I mean by this, let's make some important distinctions.

We know that *sucrose*, or table sugar, is made of glucose and fructose, two simple sugars used in the body. However, rather than providing a nourishing effect, sugar is highly addictive (Avena, Rada, and Hoebel 2008), and uses up bodily resources, such as chromium (Kozlovsky et al. 1986) and magnesium (Lemann 1976), as well as causes numerous other ill effects, such as an accelerated aging process (Lee and Cerami 1992). One recent study showed that sugar is three times as addictive as cocaine (Lenoir et al. 2007).

In the case of plant-based substances, such as wine and chocolate, there are antioxidants and other nutrients that have beneficial effects. Red wine is rich in iron and contains resveratrol, but it also contains alcohol. At a certain level, wine is a food, but above a certain threshold, it becomes a drug. Blood alcohol levels vary from one individual to the next because of differences in tolerance. The nutritive benefits of red wine are significant, but it's vital for you to know your threshold of tolerance. Both coffee and chocolate contain caffeine, which is a stimulant. In addition chocolate contains the stimulating alkaloids theophylline and theobromine, as well as the psychoactive substances anandamide and phenethylamine (Smith, Gaffan, and Rogers 2004). Stimulants like caffeine (Battram et al. 2005) and alcohol (Latenkov 1985) increase adrenaline output to excess, which eventually leads to fatigue. Both alcohol (Nurnberger and Bierut 2007) and caffeine (Juliano and Griffiths 2004) can be addictive. These nonfoods are primarily for pleasure and to alter our moods.

I taught my kids that some foods (such as ice cream and chocolate) are merely for pleasure, while other foods make us strong. Whenever I was faced with their inevitable begging for a treat, I quickly agreed but on a delayed basis. I found that even five-year-olds were willing to strike this bargain, demanding, "When Saturday comes, you'd better keep your word!" They didn't always feel well after a birthday party with lots of ice cream and cake. Rather than take a judgmental stance, I told them, "That's how Dad feels after too much ice cream."

Discerning what foods are healthy for us, and in what amounts, is a learning process. I think that using these popular less-than-nutritious foods is an important part of life, but if you need to have them every day, then you're addicted. Addiction is the archenemy of real pleasure and enjoyment. So don't tell yourself that because you're sick or overweight, or have cancer, you can never again have _____ (chocolate, a glass of wine, or whatever) again. But in time, your tastes will change so that you'll develop instincts that tell you when you can get away with eating something sweet or heavy without repercussions. You'll start to know what your body needs, because you'll train your cravings to the point where you can trust them again.

Many people have also said that they eventually reach a new intuitive level about other issues, related to their business and social lives. The five-day diet plan scrapes off your antennae and sharpens your wits. You'll also cultivate a new kind of pleasure associated with minimalism: a feeling of lightness, pleasure in small things, and appreciation of subtle flavors you weren't previously aware of. Once, during a five-day diet period, I had only juices with a few cleansing herbs and a little kelp. The day I started solid food again, I had the most urgent craving for cauliflower, of all things, which has never really been one of my favorite foods. I hungrily steamed some and drizzled a little olive oil on it. This was as unforgettable of a culinary experience as when I had eaten at a three-star restaurant in the southwest of France.

So the purpose of this "fasting with food" is not to be "good"; the purpose is empowerment. You don't give up anything, but you get a lot. You make a serious effort but not a single, sustained effort lasting for the rest of your life. Our ancestors fasted regularly. At the turn of the twentieth century, Russians fasted on water for sometimes as long as six weeks before the first day of Christmas, and broke the fast with steamed cracked wheat and honey. Most fasting periods in Western cultures conformed to the Christian calendar and were considered times of prayer and purification. The same cultures also slaughtered the fatted calf, broke out the jugs of wine, and partied heartily at festival times. I think of this as "full-spectrum living," where you learn to appreciate both fasting and feasting. In our modern culture, all we do is feast! And what do we get for it?

The five-day diet for gentle detoxification consists of the following:

> steamed vegetables and salads with small amounts of extra-virgin olive oil and vinegar (if desired)

> brown rice

> fresh juices

> fresh, seasonal fruit

Carrot-celery-apple juice is my favorite juice; I find that it helps with cravings for sweets. There are lots of juice formulas you can experiment with; for example, I also like cabbage-celery-romaine-apple juice, but other people like to add kale, a little ginger, or watercress. It's up to you. Fresh seasonal fruit is okay too.

If you're a hard-core coffee drinker, rather than stop suddenly, please taper off. You can easily cut it in half and diminish your intake gradually from there. It's important to learn how much energy you really have, not just the artificial buzz from stimulation. You can stop drinking coffee altogether if your habit is only a cup or two a day. If it's much more than that, to stop suddenly could result in severe headache, sociopathic behavior (well, at least a few mood swings), or both.

During the five-day diet, people often go through significant mood swings regardless of whether they're kicking the coffee habit. Hang in there; this is part of the learning process. Paying close attention to your bodily sensation and moods might reveal some information you can use to take charge of your life. Tell your spouse, your partner, or a friend about the diet so that you'll have an ally to rely on for emotional support. Ask your ally to remind you that emotional crises can be a part of this process. I guarantee you won't remember without a reminder, but when you're inside the emotional upheaval, a simple reminder can help take you right out of it.

Another thing to remember is that after five days, you may find yourself experiencing a particular craving, and it might not be cauliflower. It might be a cheeseburger, a pizza, chocolate, or some other type of junk food. At the end of the five-day period, I recommend indulging in anything you're craving as soon as possible. You can't go wrong. You might find that you really didn't want it after all; it just sounded good. You might find that a little bit goes a long way, that you're satisfied with a small amount. Or you might have an incredibly enhanced experience of pleasure like never before! Or perhaps not. You might feel the return or resurgence of a long-standing symptom, like an allergic reaction or a body ache. Even a painful experience will teach you something—at a deeper than intellectual level, literally at "gut" level.

Want to use herbs to assist your detoxification process? Fine! Work with a knowledgeable herbalist if you don't know much about herbs. Many health care providers use herbal detox kits or have their own approach.

I recommend using food in this diet only the first couple of periods you're on it. You can modify the diet with herbs or other supplements to suit your needs later on. The diet can be useful to improve your bodily perception and help you evaluate how various foods and supplements affect you. It's okay if you don't practice the diet perfectly the first time; you'll get another chance in a few days.

When you're not on the five-day diet, which is two thirds of the time, do the best you can. Try not to get re-addicted to any of the older habits. Don't worry about being perfect or even being "good." Give yourself a few months to get used to the diet. If you're in particularly poor health, consider drawing on your willpower to accelerate the healing process. Try to train your ally or support team to help you with the process.

## DETOXIFYING FOODS

> Sulfur-containing vegetables, such as the crucifers (cabbage family), onions, and garlic, are detoxifying (Gamet-Payrastre et al. 2000). Broccoli sprouts have an even stronger detoxifying potency than the vegetable itself (Rahman, Li, and Sarkar 2004).

> Carotene-containing vegetables, like carrots, support liver function. One very important carotene is beta-carotene, sometimes called *provitamin A*, which is another nutrient the liver needs.

> Both ginger and turmeric are anti-inflammatory. Ginger is used in botanical medicine to stimulate thyroid function, while turmeric is used in traditional herbal medicine in India and China for liver support.

> Green leafy vegetables (Gupta and Prakash 2009) and sea vegetables help remove heavy metals (Tanaka, Inoue, and Skoryna 1970).

> Psyllium-seed husks bulk the stool and help increase the volume of bowel movements.

## Water

**Water Filtration:** A reverse-osmosis system takes out bacteria, contaminants, and heavy metals, including chlorine and fluorine, that may have been added to the water supply. You don't need chlorine if there are no bacteria. You'll need to drink plenty of water during a detoxification period, at least one to two quarts a day, so it's important that it's of good quality. A carbon filter is another option, but reverse osmosis is the most thorough.

**Shower Filters:** This may seem like a bit much, but the chlorine in water turns to gas when heated and pounded against the tiles in your shower. You may be filtering chlorine out of your drinking water but absorbing it through your skin in the shower. In the shower you're exposed to twenty to twenty-five gallons of water, whereas you would drink perhaps only a quart a day.

# DEEP CLEANSING FROM ENVIRONMENTAL CHEMICALS

Chapter 7 contains more in-depth information about toxic chemicals in the environment. The Centers for Disease Control (CDC) says that 100 percent of us have toxic chemicals in our bodies, including some of the least healthful. A 2003 study by the Environmental Working Group (EWG) found that blood samples from newborns contained an average of 287 toxins, including mercury, fire retardants, pesticides, and Teflon chemicals (Environmental Working Group 2005). Almost all of these toxic chemicals can cause cancer, disrupt our hormonal systems, or both. The worst part is that we don't have the body chemistry to eliminate some of the most dangerous chemicals, like PCBs (polychlorinated biphenyl) and dioxins. As complex and diverse as they are, our metabolic chemical processes simply haven't evolved to the point where they're capable of dismantling some of these toxic molecules. These toxins accumulate in our fat and connective tissue, and even in our bones. We can't depend on the liver to detoxify them, nor can we depend on the thyroid to step up metabolism and break them down.

And what about air pollution? I can't tell you not to breathe. Of course, all this may seem pretty bleak, but the fact is, we have to live in the real world, so we may need a special strategy.

## Detoxification Nutrients for Deep Cleansing

Another area where it's good to get professional help is supplementing with nutrients that facilitate detoxification. Here are some useful supplements for maximizing the process of removing toxic materials from the body (also see the appendix):

> glutathione (an amino acid)

> alpha-lipoic acid

> garlic extracts

> hydrolyzed whey protein (food source of glutathione)

> phosphatidylcholine (found in egg yolks and lecithin)

> proteolytic enzymes (found in tropical fruits and animal organs)

> vitamin C

# How Do You Know If You Have Heavy Metals in Your Body?

Some doctors have a test that checks for heavy metals in your system. Because they may not show up in a blood test, a chemical is injected into the muscle to drive the heavy metals out of the tissues, and within twenty-four hours, the urine is checked. A simpler test, used medically and by environmental scientists for decades (see the appendix), is tissue mineral analysis, which requires taking a hair sample and testing it for toxic metals. See chapter 7 to learn more about keeping heavy metals and other toxins out of your home environment.

## SUPPLEMENTS TO HELP REMOVE HEAVY METALS FROM THE BODY

Besides far-infrared sauna treatment (discussed next), several supplements accelerate the process of removing heavy metals from the body:

> laminaria (kombu) extract

> blue-green algae (spirulina)

> modified citrus pectin

> sulfur-containing amino acids, such as glutathione, methionine, and cysteine

# Home Hyperthermia: The Far-Infrared Sauna

In chapter 2 I mentioned that because cancer cells can't stand heat, *hyperthermia*, which is actually an artificial fever, is one of the new medical technologies used in Europe and starting to be used in the United States. There's another useful role that heat can play: it can activate the tissues and stimulate the microcirculation deep in the tissues to sweat embedded toxins out through the skin, which is simply the only way to get some of these substances out of the body (Rogers 2002). You can detoxify substantially by being very active and sweating a lot. Otherwise, you can use an external heat source.

Hot-water and steam saunas and thermal spas have historically been used around the world for healing. Though saunas are powerful therapy, they're not good for people who are very sick or in a delicate condition, because the heat is too stressful for the body. Fortunately a new technology provides all of the benefits and none of the risks. Rather than heat up the whole body, the *far-infrared sauna* penetrates from one-and-a-half to two inches deep and heats connective tissue up to about 140 degrees Fahrenheit (Inoue and Kabaya 1989). Contact health care providers in your area for the availability of infrared sauna therapy, or investigate buying or building your own (see the appendix).

Is it safe? Far-infrared sauna treatment is safe even for fragile patients. Doctors at the Mayo Clinic used it with patients with advanced heart disease who were on a lot of medications. They found that the patients' conditions improved substantially, showing reduced blood pressure and fewer arrhythmias. Many of them were even able to stop taking some of their medications within three weeks. In a regular hot sauna, heart patients experienced arrhythmias but not in the far-infrared sauna (Tei and Tanaka 1996).

Does it cleanse the chemicals from the body? Scientists at the EPA showed that far-infrared sauna treatment could eliminate PCBs and other chemicals in human subjects even during their continued exposure to toxic chemicals on a daily basis (Schnare, Ben, and Shields 1984). War veterans who'd been exposed to Agent Orange experienced improvement of symptoms such as joint pain (Roehm 1983). Far-infrared sauna treatment has also successfully removed toxins from very fragile patients with severe chemical and food sensitivities (Rea et al. 1996). It can also be used to treat cancer, especially when caused by environmental toxins (Schnare and Robinson 1986).

**Additional Benefits of Far-Infrared Sauna Treatment:**

> Hyperthermia improves circulation even in the deeper areas around the abdominal organs. This relieves congestion by draining accumulated waste products from tissues throughout the body, even the coronary vessels of the heart, as studies have shown (Tei et al. 1995). This enhanced circulation results in improved oxygenation of the tissues after they're unburdened (Kihara et al. 2002).

> The sauna has a calming effect, helping to turn down the flight-or-fight sympathetic branch of the nervous system and switch on the cooling parasympathetic branch. This lowers our levels of stress hormones, thus improving immunity by allowing NK cells to become more active, an effect that's especially enhanced if you're already exercising.

> It restores electrochemical balance by removing wastes, which are mostly acidic, from the connective tissues and membranes.

> It helps water penetrate the cells and tissues.

## GUIDELINES AND SAFETY TIPS

Though this is a very safe treatment, as with any new procedure, start slowly, taking the time to get to know it. If you have high blood pressure, you may want to check your blood pressure before you enter the sauna. Also weigh yourself, because this will help determine how much fluid you lose through perspiration. Don't get in the sauna directly after a heavy meal; it's best to wait an hour or two. Start by sitting for about ten to fifteen minutes at around 100 degrees Fahrenheit to get the feel of it. Then get out of the sauna and check your blood pressure, temperature, and pulse rate. If your blood pressure has increased by 10 millimeters, body temperature has increased by over 1 degree, or pulse rate reads over 110, stop for the day. You'll gradually get used to the sauna so that you can stay in it for longer periods with fewer changes in pulse rate or blood pressure. Consider an hour a day at 140 degrees Fahrenheit to be an upper limit, but 120 degrees is plenty.

In the sauna, use towels to catch any sweat, and wipe your skin often to prevent reabsorption of toxins. Can't sweat? Try moistening the skin and covering up, if necessary. Enhancing your circulation before the sauna will also increase its efficiency, and you can do this by exercising for a few minutes or by taking niacin (discussed in the next section). If you already have a regular exercise program, it's a good idea to lighten up on that routine while establishing your sauna routine. After the sauna, take a cool or lukewarm shower, dry off, and cover up. Drink plenty of water; if your skin is wrinkled directly after the sauna or you've lost weight, you need to drink water immediately to rehydrate.

If you experience dizziness, headache, shortness of breath, rapid heart rate, weakness, cramps or spasms, or any other discomfort, discontinue the sauna for the day. Next time, start out at a lower temperature level and stay in for a shorter duration. If you don't feel well afterward, don't be discouraged. It's not a bad sign; feeling a slight malaise is just part of the detoxification process and, if experienced later in the process, could even be the result of tumor breakdown. When you experience such ill feelings, shorten your stay or turn down the heat. Since this is a very individualized process, you'll benefit from being monitored by a health care provider. But don't *expect* to feel bad; most of the time you won't. Above all, don't suffer; that's not the point. Forget about the adage, "no pain, no gain." This is your process, so it's essential to do it at your own pace.

### Detox Program Brought the Spark Back to Life

C. J., a twenty-one-year-old computer specialist, was responding poorly to chemotherapy treatment for leukemia. Exhausted from the treatment, he became unable to travel to the East Coast for work. Feeling depressed and hopeless, he saw a naturopath, who guided him through a detoxification program to complement his chemotherapy that included organic, raw and lightly cooked food, and frequent juices, along with liver-cleansing supplements. C. J.'s energy eventually returned, his outlook brightened, and his response to chemotherapy became more positive and brought his leukemia into remission.

Note that the sauna can eliminate drugs from the system faster than usual. Discuss this with your doctor if you take prescription drugs, especially blood-pressure or antiseizure medications, or hormones, such as insulin. Inform your doctor if you're pregnant or if you have metal plates in your body or a pacemaker. Don't use the sauna if you have any acute inflammation or swelling.

## SUPPLEMENTS TO USE WITH FAR-INFRARED SAUNA THERAPY

After sweating, it's important to replenish nutrients lost from your body. Obviously water is your first need, but additionally you'll need to add electrolytes lost in perspiration. Electrolytes allow the body's fluids to hold a charge in order to circulate efficiently and pass through membranes. A number of products are suitable for replacing lost electrolytes, but a simple solution is to take kelp tablets or laminaria (a sea vegetable, also called "kombu") extract (Kolb et al. 2004). Specific minerals, such as magnesium, may need to be replaced, especially if you experience muscle cramps or spasms, or an irregular heartbeat. Magnesium is usually insufficient in the diet and gets leached out easily by sugar and alcohol (Lemann 1976). The form of magnesium is important, because some forms can cause bowel rumbling (see the appendix). With prostate cancer, zinc is always important as well. Another quick and easy solution is Emergen-C, available at natural-food stores and other stores. You may want to use two or three packets in up to a quart of water if you've had a good sweat. Most people can take a daily dose of up to 5 grams of vitamin C, but if you have diarrhea or bowel rumbling, find a lower dose that you can tolerate, starting at around 500 milligrams (Cathcart 1981). Weigh yourself, and if you've lost weight during the sauna session, replace that water. A gallon of water weighs about eight pounds.

*Niacin* (vitamin B3) causes flushing, which, though temporarily uncomfortable, stimulates metabolism and opens up deep circulation. Start with a dose of about 100 milligrams. Don't get into the sauna until the flushing settles down. You can gradually increase your niacin intake, in increments of 50 to 100 milligrams, as your tolerance increases. Some people take as much as 2,000 milligrams, but most people can work up to around 500 milligrams. In medical studies on using niacin for treatment of cardiovascular and other disorders, 1,500 milligrams was considered a low dose (Gardner et al. 1997).

---

# SYMPTOMS NECESSITATING REGULAR DETOXIFICATION

Circle "Y" for yes or "N" for no, and mark in one point for each yes answer unless otherwise noted:

Y or N  _____  Do you feel faint or dizzy when it's time to eat?

Y or N  _____  Are you hungry all the time?

Y or N    _____    Do you have a good appetite?

Y or N    _____    Do you feel as if food just sits in your stomach?

Y or N    _____    Do you have any food allergies or intolerances?

Y or N    _____    Do you often have acid reflux (stomach acid rising up the esophagus, causing a burning discomfort)?

Y or N    _____    Do you crave fats or heavy food with each meal?

Y or N    _____    Do you feel tired after eating?

Y or N    _____    Do you eat sugar every day?

Y or N    _____    Do you drink colas or other soft drinks? If so, how often (two points = every day, one = three or fewer times a week)?

Y or N    _____    Do you drink alcohol more than three times a week (two points if you drink spirits daily)?

Y or N    _____    Do you get migraines one or more times a month, or tension headaches one or more times a week?

Y or N    _____    Do you have chronic neck or back tightness or pain?

Y or N    _____    Do you have hemorrhoids?

Y or N    _____    Do you experience bleeding gums or other gum problems?

Y or N    _____    Do you experience premenstrual mood swings?

Y or N    _____    Do you get menstrual cramps?

Y or N    _____    Do you experience menopausal depression or mood swings?

Y or N    _____    Do you experience menopausal anxiety or panic attacks?

Y or N    _____    Do you drink coffee every day? If so, how many cups (add a point for more than two cups a day)?

Y or N    _____    Do you usually feel mentally alert and clear (if no, add a point)?

Y or N    _____    Do you take any prescription drugs daily?

If you scored over five points, you're in the majority. Consider a detoxification program, but take it easy at first and be sure to get professional support.

At the risk of appearing contradictory, I feel it's important to state that being too rigid can jeopardize your success with changing your lifestyle. You need to exercise good judgment and use strict discipline during your five-day-diet periods, but it's important to relax a bit after that. It's okay to enjoy coffee, tea, chocolate and other sweets, and alcohol. Enjoyment is *good* for you, and will also give you a chance to see if indulging in these addictive foods really enhances your well-being or if you can enjoy smaller quantities of them than before. Understand that the purpose of the five-day diet is to help you to *avoid* having to give up the things you love and to make sure that they don't hurt you or interfere with your longevity and well-being. A detoxification program may not cure any or all of the symptoms mentioned in the previous questionnaire or make an immediate difference, but those complaints usually improve.

# CHAPTER 5

# Cancer-Fighting Foods

Diet is the most important lifestyle change you can make to build immunity and strength. As we all know, improving the diet is about looking and feeling better, but as you'll see, it's also about changing the body's chemistry down to the cellular level. You'll see how different foods can prevent the formation of cancer cells and improve the body's efficiency in getting rid of them. Remember from chapter 1, we all produce abnormal cells and have several mechanisms to get rid of them. This chapter discusses how to do this on a daily basis. You've also learned that cancer rates have increased dramatically in recent decades. Radiation and toxic chemicals in the environment are important factors, but the most important factor is probably what most of us do three times a day with our food consumption. The mainstream scientific community first identified the link between cancer and diet in the 1970s (National Academy of Sciences 1982), and today there's enough scientific evidence to enable us to fine-tune our diets to reduce our risk and improve our health, even if we already have cancer (World Cancer Research Fund 2009). The National Cancer Institute has supported a cancer chemoprevention program called Natural Inhibitors of Carcinogenesis (1991 to 2004) in laboratories at the University of Illinois, Chicago, and Purdue University. These researchers have collaborated with other researchers internationally to find new cancer chemopreventive agents from plants, particularly edible ones (Natural Inhibitors of Carcinogenesis Project, http://nic.pharmacy.purdue.edu).

# CANCER-PROMOTING FOODS

Recent investigation into the average Western diet reveals that about 56 percent of its calories come from three categories (Cordain et al. 2005):

> ➤ sugars (such as cane sugar, corn syrup, and fructose)

> ➤ white flour (such as white bread and refined pasta) and white rice

> ➤ vegetable oils (such as soy, sunflower, corn, and hydrogenated oils)

These sources, however, contain very little protein, vitamins, minerals, or omega-3 fatty acids, which are all essential for the body's health. These foods directly stimulate and nourish the growth of cancer (Michaud et al. 2002).

## Sugar and White Flour

Dr. Otto Warburg won the Nobel Prize in Physiology or Medicine for his discovery that tumors depend on glucose (the form of sugar that's in the blood and is used by the tissues) as the main source of fuel. The PET scan, which, as previously mentioned, is one of today's methods of detecting cancer, measures the body's metabolism of glucose. The scan highlights areas in the body that consume a lot of glucose and identifies them as places where there's a high probability of cancer. If we consume a lot of sugar, white flour, or anything containing carbohydrates (see table 5.1), the body immediately releases insulin to help glucose penetrate the cells. Another substance, *IGF-1 (insulin-like growth factor 1)*, accompanies insulin and also has the property of stimulating cell growth. In addition to rapid cell growth, insulin and IGF-1 promote inflammation (Rajpathak et al. 2008). As you learned in chapter 1, inflammation sets the stage for the tumor growth. Today we know that insulin and IGF-1 not only stimulate growth of cancer cells but also the ability of abnormal cells to invade surrounding tissues (Dunn et al. 1997). We also know that diabetics (who have excessively high levels of glucose in the blood) have a higher than average risk of developing cancer (Weiderpass et al. 1997). Scientific research has established this adverse relationship between several types of cancer and high insulin levels. In men, the risk of developing prostate cancer is nine times higher with abnormally high levels of IGF-1 (Chan et al. 1998). A high glycemic diet, high in fast-burning sugars and starches, is also associated with ovarian (Augustin et al. 2003), pancreatic (Michaud et al. 2002), and colon cancers (Franceschi et al. 2001).

All of this research implies that drastic limitation of sugar and white flour intake is important to prevent cancer and its recurrence or improve the chances of a favorable response to cancer treatment. Eating sweets between meals seems to have the most damaging effect, because there's nothing to slow down the sudden rise in insulin. Fruits and vegetables, which contain fiber, and healthy oils, like olive oil and butter, can act as a buffer and offset increased insulin caused by simple sugars. Later in this chapter you'll learn that there are foods that reduce the level of sugar in the blood.

## TABLE 5.1 GLYCEMIC SCALE

(Foster-Powell, Holt, and Brand-Miller 2002)

| High Glycemic (Reduce or Eliminate) | Low Glycemic (Choose) |
|---|---|
| ➤ Sugars: white, raw, evaporated cane juice, corn syrup (including high-fructose corn syrup), maple syrup, dextrose, honey<br><br>➤ White flour, white bread, white rice, pasta, sweetened morning breakfast cereals<br><br>➤ Jams, sweetened fruits, fruits in syrup<br><br>➤ Soft drinks, commercial fruit juices | ➤ Agave syrup, malt syrup, xylitol<br><br>➤ Whole grains, brown rice, multigrain bread, spelt bread, whole grain and multigrain pastas<br><br>➤ Sweet potatoes, yams, lentils, peas, green beans, oats, muesli<br><br>➤ Fruit, especially cherries, raspberries, and blueberries<br><br>➤ Filtered water with fruits or herbs, raw juices, green tea, unsweetened grain or nut milks<br><br>➤ Burdock, fenugreek, onions, shallots, (Duraffourd and Lapraz 2002) and garlic (Thomson et al. 2006) (these foods have blood-sugar stabilizing properties) |

## Excess Omega-6 Fatty Acids

One fundamental change in diet that's occurred wasn't widely known until recent years (Ailhaud and Guesnet 2004): the shift away from a diet balanced between omega-3 and omega-6 fatty acids. Traditional diets as diverse as those of the Japanese and the natives of Greenland con-

## Body Weight and Cancer Risk

A combined analysis of 221 studies on the relationship between cancer and body weight, reviewing over 250,000 cases of cancer, revealed that risk is increased not only in common cancers, such as breast, bowel, and kidney, but also in less common cancers, such as blood cancers (for example, myeloma and leukemia) and skin cancers (such as melanoma). In women, an increase in body mass increased the risk of esophageal cancer by 51 percent, kidney cancer by 34 percent, and endometrial and gallbladder cancer by 59 percent each. In men, increased body mass raised the risk of esophageal cancer by 52 percent, thyroid cancer by 33 percent, and colon and kidney cancers each by 24 percent (Renehan et al. 2008).

Apart from increasing cancer risk, obesity is considered to be the cause of over 300,000 deaths per year and has overtaken tobacco smoking as the main preventable cause of illness and premature death since 2005. Fat consumption may not be as significant a factor in weight gain as the *types* of fats consumed. Even though fat consumption by Americans decreased 1 percent and overall calorie intake by 4 percent between 1976 and 2000, the obesity rate increased by 31 percent. This is a well-established fact, sometimes referred to as "the American Paradox" (Heini and Weinsier 1997).

Even more puzzling is the fact that the amount of fat tissue in infants less than one year old *doubled* between the years 1970 and 1990. Infants can't be accused of gorging on junk food at fast-food restaurants, constantly snacking, or being couch potatoes. Researchers have suggested that the quantity of mother's milk hasn't changed since 1950, but the *quality* has changed considerably (Ailhaud and Guesnet 2004).

tained close to equal quantities of these fatty acids (Kromann and Green 1980). Today the quantity of omega-6 fatty acids far exceeds that of omega-3 fatty acids. Taking in both types is essential, because our bodies can't manufacture them. However, their effects on the body are opposite: omega-6 fatty acids promote fat storage, blood coagulation, and an inflammatory response (Simopoulos 1999), whereas omega-3 fatty acids calm inflammation (Endres et al. 1989) and the nervous system, build brain and nervous-system tissue (Innis 2007), and reduce fat-cell production (Okuno et al. 1997). Instead of having an approximately equal amount of omega-3 and omega-6 fatty acids in our diet, we get an excess of omega-6 in a ratio of 15 to 1 (Kiecolt-Glaser et al. 2007). Our genetic patterns were established on a ratio of 1 to 1 (Simopoulos 2008). Both types of fatty acids play necessary roles in maintaining health, but an imbalance can cause health problems, as many recent studies have shown (Simopoulos 2002).

The main cause of this excess of omega-6 is changes in the diets of the livestock in our food chain. Farm animals, especially cattle and chickens, were once allowed to free-range feed; that is, cattle ate grass and herbs in the fields, and chickens, being omnivores, foraged for herbs and insects throughout the farm. Livestock are now fed a diet rich in corn and soybeans, and produce meat, milk, and eggs that are rich in omega-6 fatty acids. Eggs from chickens raised on corn contain twenty times more omega-6 than omega-3 fatty acids, but in eggs from free-range chickens, they're approximately equal (Weill et al. 2002).

# TABLE 5.2 EFFECTS OF OMEGA-3 AND OMEGA-6 FATTY ACIDS

| Omega-6 | Omega-3 |
|---|---|
| Causes inflammation | Fights inflammation |
| Coagulates blood | Thins blood |
| Stimulates cell growth | Controls cell growth |

Reduced consumption of fish can cause hormonal imbalance (discussed next). Many fish are extremely rich, not only in omega-3 fatty acids but also in other factors important for brain and nervous-system health. The problem with seafood consumption is the possible presence of mercury contaminants, but it's possible to reduce this risk by consuming fish known to have less accumulated mercury. There are also measures we can take to help eliminate mercury from the body, such as taking laminaria extract, which, as previously mentioned, is a sea vegetable product that absorbs heavy metals and other toxic substances in the intestine (Tanaka, Inoue, and Skoryna 1970). Modified citrus pectin is another plant-derived substance for detoxifying heavy metals from the system (Eliaz et al. 2006).

## Hormones

Hormones are another cause of adverse changes in the quality of our supply of animal protein. Estrogen-like hormones, such as estradiol and zeranol (banned by the European Union) (Scientific Committee on Veterinary Measures Relating to Public Health 1999), fatten up farm animals but also have negative effects that transfer to the consumer (Kart et al. 2008). *Recombinant bovine growth hormone* (*rBGH*) (banned in Europe and Canada) is a genetically engineered hormone injected into lactating cows to make them produce more milk. It promotes the cow's production of IGF-1, which is then found in the milk and, since it survives pasteurization, finds its way into the consumer. As discussed, IGF-1 is a major stimulant of fat-cell production and may even directly accelerate tumor growth.

## Trans Fats: The Worst of All

*Trans fat* is the popular name for fats that have been partially hydrogenated so that oils remain solid at warmer temperatures. Raising the melting point made it possible to create butter substitutes, and also gave the oils a longer shelf life. The problem is that trans fats increase the risk of coronary heart disease (Mozaffarian et al. 2006). Scientists believe that humans lack an enzyme for breaking trans fats down efficiently, which causes them to remain in the blood longer than other fats (Kleiman et al. 1970). As for cancer risk, the concern is that trans fats promote inflammation (Lopez-Garcia et al. 2005). There's also a possible link between trans fat consumption and prostate cancer risk (Chavarro et al. 2006). Trans fats also promote weight gain. In groups consuming the same number of calories, people who ate trans fats gained more weight (Gosline 2006). Trans fats are found in fried foods, like french fries and doughnuts, and most commercially baked goods, like pastries, pie crusts, biscuits, pizza dough, cookies, crackers, margarine, and shortening. You can tell if a food contains trans fats if the ingredient list contains "partially hydrogenated oils."

In a nutshell, cancer-promoting foods, which you'll want to decrease or avoid, are as follows:

➤ simple sugars and white flour

➤ omega-6 fatty acids

➤ animal products from livestock injected with hormones

➤ all trans (hydrogenated) fats

## TABLE 5.3 FOODS AND CANCER

| Cancer-Promoting Foods | Cancer-Fighting Foods |
|---|---|
| ➤ Foods high on the glycemic index | ➤ Fruits, grains low on the glycemic index |
| ➤ Hydrogenated or partially hydrogenated oils | ➤ Olive oil |
| ➤ Conventional dairy products (high in omega-6 fatty acids) | ➤ Butter from grass-fed cows |
| ➤ Fried foods, potato chips, corn chips | ➤ Macadamia nut oil |
| ➤ Red meat, unless free range (high in omega-6 fatty acids) | ➤ Coconut oil |
| ➤ Poultry, unless free range (high omega-6 fatty acids) | ➤ Almond milk |
| ➤ Fruit and vegetable peels, if not organic | ➤ Olives |
| ➤ Tap water (Cantor et al. 1998) | ➤ Hummus |
| | ➤ Multigrain bread |
| | ➤ Fruits and vegetables peeled and washed, if not organic |
| | ➤ Tap water filtered by reverse osmosis |

# FOODS THAT FIGHT CANCER

Rule number one is to eat organic foods and free-range or grass-fed animal products. Eliminating environmental toxins from our bodies is much more difficult when toxins accumulate several times a day. Rule number two is to minimize animal protein altogether. This doesn't mean that meat is necessarily bad for you, but in the past, people seldom ate large amounts of meat day after day. Use meats more as a condiment. Think of the classic pork and beans: a little pork or bacon was used to help flavor and enrich the beans. Also consider a stir-fry: a little meat with a lot of vegetables, including sprouts, flash-cooked so that the inside of the vegetables is warm, but they're still crisp and rich in natural enzymes. Cheeses were also used in a supplementary fashion and were often served at the end of meals, sometimes with fruit. Used in this way, a food like cheese that's rich in friendly bacteria (probiotics) and enzymes helps aid digestion of the meal. See tables 5.1 and 5. 3 for help with this strategy. While there's no perfect diet for everyone, taking foods from each category will cover not only your body's structural needs, such as replacing cells and tissues, but also the needs of the immune system and general metabolism. When these needs aren't met, we set the stage for illness, weight gain, and blood-sugar disorders, as well as serious threats like cancer.

## TABLE 5.4 DIETARY RECOMMENDATIONS

| Animal Proteins (Optional) | Whole Grains | Fats | Herbs & Spices | Vegetables & Fruits |
|---|---|---|---|---|
| ➤ Fish<br><br>➤ Free-range meat<br><br>➤ Organic eggs (of free-range chickens)<br><br>➤ Omega-3 eggs | ➤ Brown rice<br><br>➤ Millet<br><br>➤ Multigrain bread<br><br>➤ Spelt<br><br>➤ Oats<br><br>➤ Bulgur<br><br>➤ Flaxseeds | ➤ Olive oil<br><br>➤ Macadamia nut oil<br><br>➤ Butter from grass-fed cows<br><br>➤ Raw milk cheeses | ➤ Turmeric<br><br>➤ Thyme<br><br>➤ Rosemary<br><br>➤ Ginger<br><br>➤ Garlic<br><br>➤ Parsley | ➤ Crucifers<br><br>➤ Lentils<br><br>➤ Peas<br><br>➤ Beans:<br>chick peas<br>adzuki<br>black turtle<br>chili beans<br><br>➤ Sea vegetables<br><br>➤ Mushrooms<br><br>➤ Root vegetables:<br>carrot<br>turnip<br>daikon<br>parsnip<br><br>➤ Fruits:<br>berries<br>papaya<br>mango |

# Why Eat Organic?

Since the Second World War, we've lived in a different world. The annual production of synthetic chemicals exceeded 1 million tons in 1930 compared to 200 million tons today (Davis and Magee 1979). Many of these chemicals accumulate in the environment, and some of them in our bodies. We've also seen the dawn of a type of medical practice that's almost completely dependent on synthetic pharmaceutical drugs for treatment of disease. Food production methods also changed during this period such that food that's not contaminated with chemicals was given a new name: *organic*.

Organic food must comply with strict standards regulated by the federal government. An organic farm must be free of prohibited chemicals for at least three years and submit an "Organic Systems Plan" that excludes the use of synthetic chemicals and drugs with any seeds, soil, crops, or animals. The plan must include access to outdoors for animals and access to pasture for ruminants (grass and leaf-eating animals that chew a cud), and must comply with numerous other regulations (Baker et al. 2005).

A major study funded by the European Union (Taylor 2007) concluded that organic food is more nutritious than ordinary commercial produce. They found that organic fruits and vegetables had up to 40 percent more antioxidants than produce grown using pesticides. Organic produce was also shown to have higher levels of key minerals, such as iron and zinc. Levels of antioxidants in milk from organic cattle were an incredible 50 to 80 percent higher than in regular commercial milk. Researchers from the University of California (UC), Davis, found that organically grown kiwifruit had 17 percent more polyphenols (discussed later in this chapter) and 14 percent more vitamin C (ibid.). In another UC study (ibid.), researchers found that organic tomatoes contain almost twice as much quercetin and kaempferol, two important *flavonoids* (plant nutrients that are water-soluble pigments; also called *bioflavonoids*, they're considered to have antioxidant and anti-inflammatory properties).

## TABLE 5.5 VEGETABLES AND FRUITS WITH HIGHEST AND LOWEST PESTICIDE-CONTAMINATION LEVELS

(Adapted from Environmental Working Group, www.foodnews.org/fulllist.php)

Ranked on a scale from 1 to 100 according to criteria including percentage of samples with pesticides, number of pesticides on samples, and quantity of pesticides in samples.

| Highest Levels (Except Organic) | Lowest Levels |
|---|---|
| 100–30 (most contaminated to least; for example, peaches are the most contaminated) | 0–30 (least contaminated to most; for example, onions are the least contaminated) |
| Peach | Onion |
| Apple | Avocado |
| Sweet bell pepper | Sweet corn (frozen) |
| Celery | Pineapple |
| Nectarine | Mango |
| Strawberries | Asparagus |
| Cherries | Sweet peas (frozen) |
| Kale | Kiwi |
| Lettuce | Cabbage |
| Grapes (imported) | Eggplant |
| Carrot | Papaya |
| Pear | Watermelon |
| Collard greens | Broccoli |
| Spinach | Tomato |
| Potato | Sweet potato |
| Green beans | Grapefruit |
| Summer squash | Honeydew melon |
| Pepper | |
| Cucumber | |
| Raspberries | |
| Grapes (domestic) | |
| Plum | |
| Orange | |
| Cauliflower | |
| Tangerine | |
| Mushrooms | |
| Banana | |
| Winter squash | |
| Cantaloupe | |
| Cranberries | |

## What About Meat?

Heavy protein foods, like meats and cheeses, are best digested during the day, such as in the morning or afternoon, because there's a daily rhythm for converting proteins into activating substances, such as the hormone adrenaline (Ehret et al. 1999). The body stores the substances it needs from proteins until they're necessary later on for the night cycle (Fernstrom et al. 1979). In the evening, have a light meal with complex carbohydrates, such as rice and seasonal vegetables or salads. The body needs carbohydrates in the evening to support the nighttime body chemistry devoted to repair, healing, and detoxification (Adam and Oswald 1983). If you do this for only a few days, you'll feel the difference when you wake up in the morning. Preparing meat in advance by marinating it with herbs, such as thyme and rosemary, along with garlic, onions, and even red wine, improves health benefits and digestibility (Smith, Ameri, and Gadgil 2008) as well as flavor.

An important ingredient for not only meat dishes but also all kinds of soups and even vegetable dishes is stock. Stocks have minerals and nutrients from the animal's bones, connective tissue, and gelatin. Our ancestors used the entire animal in stocks. The head and hooves were once the most expensive parts because of the gelatin content. You can make stocks with bones and cartilage of grass-fed beef or free-range chicken by simmering with vegetables and herbs (as a bouquet garni) for several hours (thirty-six hours for beef because of the large bones, and eight hours for chicken or turkey) and straining. You can freeze the stock for up to three months and use it not only to add flavor to other dishes but also to make them more nutritious. You'll find that meals are more satisfying and stocks "stretch" a small amount of meat into a satisfying meal.

## TABLE 5.6 PRINCIPAL SOURCES OF OMEGA-3 FATTY ACIDS

Grams of Omega-3 Fatty Acids per 100 Gram Serving

| | |
|---|---|
| Clam (softshell) | 0.4 |
| Cod (Atlantic) | 0.3 |
| Cod (Pacific) | 0.2 |
| Crab | 0.3–0.4 |
| Eel (wild) | 0.9 |
| Haddock | 0.2 |
| Halibut | 0.5–0.9 |
| Herring (Atlantic) | 1.7 |
| Herring (Pacific) | 1.8 |
| Lobster | 0.3 |
| Mackerel (Atlantic) | 2.6 |
| Oysters (Atlantic) | 0.4 |
| Oysters (Pacific) | 0.6 |
| Salmon (different varieties of wild) | 1.0–1.5 |
| Sardines | 1.4 |
| Scallop | 0.2 |
| Sole | 0.1 |
| Trout (lake) | 2.0 |
| Trout (rainbow) | 0.6 |
| Tuna, albacore | 1.5 |
| Tuna, bluefin | 1.6 |
| Tuna, skipjack | 0.4 |

Source: USDA, Human Nutrition Information Service

# Fats and Oils

Balancing your intake of omega-6 and omega-3 fatty acids is crucial. Good sources of omega-3 oils are fish oils. Numerous fish oils are on the market, but it's best to find one that's refrigerated, guaranteed to be free of mercury, and preferably preserved with vitamin E to ensure freshness. An easy-to-digest oil is krill oil, which is an excellent source of omega-3s that's also rich in antioxidants. A staple of the Mediterranean diet, extra-virgin olive oil is one of the best oils for health. Olive oil has a low smoke point, however, and isn't as good for sautéing, since it oxidizes at a low temperature. Olive oil is rich in monounsaturated fatty acids, which are believed to offer protection against certain cancers, such as breast (Simonsen et al. 1998) and colon cancer (Stoneham et al. 2000). Monounsaturated fats are typically high in vitamin E, the antioxidant vitamin that's usually in short supply in many Western diets (Ahuja, Goldman, and Moshfegh 2004). Foods rich in monounsaturates are easy to assimilate. Macadamia nut oil, macadamia nuts, and avocados are also rich sources. Oils to avoid or consume in limited quantity are corn, soy, safflower, peanut, sesame, and cottonseed because of their high omega-6 fatty acid content. Canola oil is controversial because it's highly processed. The omega-3 fatty acids convert to trans fats (O'Keefe et al. 1994). Saturated fats, also necessary to the diet, are found not only in butter, cheese, and other animal fats, but also in unrefined, organic coconut oil.

## TABLE 5.7 FISH WITH HIGHEST MERCURY LEVELS

**Highest Levels:**
Shark
Swordfish
King mackerel

**Lower Levels:**
Anchovies
Butterfish
Catfish
Clam
Cod
Crab
Crawfish
Haddock (Atlantic)
Herring
Jacksmelt
Lobster (spiny)
Mackerel Atlantic (N. Atlantic)
Mackerel, chub (Pacific)
Mullet
Oyster
Perch (ocean)
Pollock
Salmon (canned)
Salmon (fresh and frozen)
Sardine
Scallop
Shad American
Shrimp
Squid
Tilapia
Trout (freshwater)
Tuna (canned, light)
Whitefish

Source: U.S. Food and Drug Administration 2006

## FLAXSEEDS

Flaxseeds are a rich source of omega-3 fatty acids. However, the oil is unstable and oxidizes easily, so it's best to grind the seeds and use in food or a smoothie. Using the seeds also allows you to get the lignans, substances with cancer-preventing properties, which aren't available in the oil; fiber is also available only in the seeds. Keep the oil refrigerated and use it cold rather than cooking with it. Poultry fed a diet including flaxseeds lay eggs that are rich in omega-3 fatty acids. In a study at Duke University, daily consumption of 30 grams of flaxseeds slowed down the growth of prostate cancer from 30 to 40 percent, because it apparently blocks angiogenesis (Demark-Wahnefried et al. 2001).

## CLA FROM GRASS-FED ANIMALS

Another important anticancer component in food comes from animal fat: CLA (*conjugated linoleic acid*) is a fatty acid that has a direct role in suppressing cancer cells, and it's found in meat and dairy products of animals that were fed grass and herbs. Grazing animals have three to five times more CLA than animals fattened on grain in a feedlot (Garton 1960). Simply switching from products of grain-fed animals to those of grass-fed ones can greatly increase your intake of CLA (Kraft et al. 2008). Small amounts of CLA have blocked all three stages of cancer: initiation, promotion, and metastasis, whereas most anticancer agents block only one of these stages (Ip, Scimeca, and Thompson 1994). What's more, CLA has slowed the growth of an unusually wide variety of tumors, including skin, breast, prostate, and colon cancers (ibid.). A recent survey determined that women with the most CLA in their diets had a 60 percent reduction in the risk of breast cancer (Aro et al. 2000). CLA also may restrict weight gain (Miner et al. 2001). I don't recommend using a synthetic CLA supplement because of evidence that it may cause liver swelling and insulin resistance; it's much better to get CLA in the amounts available in grass-fed animals (Larsen, Toubro, and Astrup 2003).

# Green Tea

Green tea is rich in chemicals called *polyphenols*, antioxidants that reduce inflammation and improve blood circulation by lowering bad cholesterol. In green tea a polyphenol called *EGCG* (*epigallocatechin 3-gallate*) reduces the growth of new blood vessels (angiogenesis) (Cao and Cao 1999), which are essential to tumor growth and metastasis. (Another important polyphenol, called *resveratrol*, found in red wine, also has anti-inflammatory properties [Manna, Mukhopadhyay, and Aggarwal 2000].) EGCG also activates liver enzymes to improve detoxification (Goodin and Rosengren 2003). For the best result, steep the tea for eight minutes or longer to extract all of the polyphenols. Five to six cups a day provide a sufficient dose of these important nutrients. If you're caffeine sensitive, decaffeinated green tea still contains all of the polyphenols. Black tea is from the same plant as green tea, but it's fermented, which destroys most of the polyphenols.

## Garlic and Onion Family

Garlic has antioxidant effects and also induces apoptosis (cell death) in cancer cells in colon, breast, lung, and prostate cancer and in leukemia (Hsing et al. 2002). Garlic is used in medical herbalism in Europe to stimulate the thyroid and to deter bacterial growth. Louis Pasteur observed garlic's antibacterial effect in 1858 (Pasteur 1858). Garlic was used as a wound disinfectant in World Wars I and II. In the Second World War, garlic was called "Russian penicillin," because the Russians had to use it when they ran low on regular antibiotics. In addition, all of the vegetables of the onion family regulate blood sugar by reducing the amount of insulin and IGF-1, thereby inhibiting cancer-cell growth (Thomson and Ali 2003). Garlic is most effective when crushed into olive oil so that volatile oils dissolve in the olive oil and don't escape. You can consume garlic and onions cooked or raw. Some of the garlic supplement products don't contain all of the active chemicals in raw garlic (Lawson and Wang 2001).

## Crucifers

The crucifers of the brassica family are cabbages, kale, broccoli, brussels sprouts, and cauliflower. The protective effect of brassicas against cancer is probably due to their relatively high content of glucosinolates and indole-3-carbinols, both of which have shown anticancer properties (van Poppel et al. 1999). The crucifers interfere with the ability of precancerous cells to form malignant tumors, and they also promote cancer-cell apoptosis and block angiogenesis. Overcooking crucifers can destroy some of these active chemical components, so it's best to eat them lightly steamed or raw. In a study of 29,000 men over a four-year period, those who consumed more than one serving per week of cruciferous vegetables reduced their risk of prostate cancer by 59 percent (Kirsh et al. 2007). Cruciferous vegetables outside the brassica family include arugula, radish, watercress, daikon radish, and horseradish, which also have cancer preventive properties (Keck and Finley 2004).

## Carotenes

Carotenes are a large group of red and yellow plant pigments that are vital for the photosynthesis process, and protect the plant against damage from the free radicals produced during photosynthesis. Carotenes are found in carrots, sweet potatoes, zucchini, pumpkins, tomatoes, apricots, and beets, as well as all fruits and vegetables with red, yellow, and orange pigments. The vitamin A found in colorful fruits and vegetables is called *provitamin A carotenoid*. Vitamin A is an essential nutrient for the liver. One of the carotenes, lycopene, inhibits cancer cells, even some of the most virulent ones, like glioma brain cells (Sharoni, Danilenko, and Levy 2000). Carotenes, such as lycopene, lutein, canthaxanthin, astaxanthine, and others, stimulate the immune system to activate the NK cells. Research has shown that women with breast cancer who consume more carotene-rich foods live longer than those who don't eat as many such foods (Ingram 1994). Beta-carotene is probably the best known of the carotenoids, those red, orange, and yellow pigments that give color to many fruits and vegetables. The body converts beta-carotene into vitamin A. Carrots and beets contain large amounts of beta-carotene. Taken as a supplement, this powerful antioxidant counters the effects of free radicals and may help to protect against and treat certain cancers (Peto et al. 1981).

## TOMATOES

The lycopene in tomatoes is known to increase survival in men with prostate cancer who consume tomato sauce at least twice a week (Chan et al. 2006). Lycopene is more available to the body if the tomatoes are cooked with a certain amount of fat, such as from olive oil (Sies and Stahl 1998).

## Turmeric

Because turmeric is a yellow powdered herb, it's the most conspicuous ingredient in curry powder, but it's also used as a medicinal herb in Ayurvedic and Chinese medicine. It's used to promote bile flow and as a potent anti-inflammatory agent that helps prevent development of cancer cells. It stimulates liver detoxification of carcinogens (Goud, Polasa, and Krishnaswamy 1993), induces apoptosis of cancer cells (Chakravarty and Yasmin 2005), and inhibits angiogenesis (Mohan et al. 2000). Turmeric inhibits the growth of many types of cancer, including breast, ovarian, colon, liver, and stomach cancers (Aggarwal, Kumar, and Bharti 2003), as well as leukemia (Nagabhushan and Bhide 1992). In laboratory studies, it increased the effectiveness of chemotherapy in tumor destruction. People in India eat around 2 grams of turmeric a day, which might be one reason why they have a lower cancer risk. The curcumin in turmeric was found to make glioblastoma (a type of brain cancer) cells more sensitive to chemotherapy (Gao et al. 2005). Researchers speculate that one way it works is to suppress NF-$k$B (introduced in chapter 1), which protects cancer cells from the body's natural defenses (Shishodia et al. 2005). Turmeric is absorbed much more efficiently if mixed with black pepper (Shoba et al. 1998), and you can use it as a condiment in sauces over meat or vegetables.

## Ginger

Ginger is another herb that's used in Chinese medicine, Ayurvedic medicine, and Western herbalism for various healing purposes. It's good for nausea and dissolves phlegm that has accumulated in the gastrointestinal tract (Bone et al. 1990), and Western herbalism employs it to stimulate the thyroid, to reduce fever, to strengthen immunity, and to relieve lung congestion.

Ginger is also a powerful anti-inflammatory and antioxidant, and it prevents tumors from forming new blood vessels (Kikuzaki and Nakatani 1993).

## Mushrooms

In recent years many types of mushrooms—shiitake, maitake, reishi, portobello, and others—have been studied for their immune-boosting properties (Ooi and Liu 2000). In Japan mushroom extracts are used in cancer treatment to support the immune system. Japanese researchers (Hara et al. 2003) found that people who ate a lot of mushrooms, like shiitake, had half the rate of stomach cancer as those who didn't eat them. Though mushrooms are a part of the Japanese diet, several mushroom products specially designed to enhance immunity have been developed for medical use, especially for cancer treatment (Matsui et al. 2002). Fermentation enhances the benefits of these mushrooms, because some of the molecules that are active in supporting the immune system, such as beta-glucan, are very large. Fermentation breaks these molecules down into smaller, more absorbable components and creates new ones that are even more active in building immunity (Smith, Rowan, and Sullivan 2002).

## Soy Products

Soy products are the subject of some controversy because of their well-known estrogen-like properties. Since estrogen is fuel for most cancers (Cavalieri et al. 1997), we should avoid foods containing it at all costs. However, it's true that the phytoestrogens in soy are less biologically active than the estrogens the body produces. Soy-based medications are used for prostate cancer prevention (Davis et al. 2000), but many cancers might be caused at least partially by estrogen-mimicking chemicals in the environment called *xenoestrogens* (Fernandez et al. 2008). For people who actually have cancer, especially women with breast cancer or one of the reproductive cancers, soy-derived products have powerful therapeutic properties. In such cases, it's best to work with a health care provider who's experienced in their use.

Fairly difficult to digest, soy protein is controversial as a health food. This is true of both tofu and commercial, industrial soy proteins used as food additives. Tofu is usually served hot in Japan, with a small amount of soy sauce and raw, grated ginger on top to help digest it. On the other hand, fermented products, like miso, don't have this estrogenic quality. Miso, a salty soybean paste that's fermented and aged for months or years, is an excellent food for building strength and for encouraging healthy bacterial proliferation in the gastrointestinal flora. You can serve it by stirring it into hot water (but don't boil it or you'll kill the friendly microbes), but it tastes best when stirred into fish stock. Vegetarians serve it in a vegetable or seaweed stock. Japanese people often start the day with a bowl of miso soup. Excellent for a sensitive stomach, miso also helps with digestion after you've overeaten.

# Seaweeds

A staple in the Japanese diet, seaweeds are also found in Southeast Asian and the Mediterranean diets. The most common edible seaweeds are nori (used in sushi rolls), kombu, wakame, arame, and dulse. Seaweeds can provide trace minerals that are otherwise hard to get, because they're rich in minerals from the sea and have nourishing, alkalizing, and detoxifying properties. Research shows that molecules in seaweeds inhibit the growth of cancer cells, in particular breast, prostate, colon, and skin cancers (Maruyama et al. 2003). Fucoidan, found in kombu (laminaria) and wakame, causes apoptosis of cancer cells and stimulates immunity, for example, the activity of NK cells. Another component of kombu, *fucoxanthin* is a carotenoid, like beta-carotene or lycopene, yet it's stronger than lycopene in inhibiting cancer-cell growth (Shimizu et al. 2005). Seaweeds also contain *alginates*, salts of alginic acid that form a viscous, gelatinous substance that has the ability to absorb toxic materials, even toxic metals like mercury, from the intestines.

# Fruits

Several fruits, especially blueberries, bilberries, raspberries, cranberries, pomegranates, cherries, strawberries, and blackberries, are rich in polyphenols, including one called *ellagic acid*, which is also found in walnuts and pecans. All polyphenols inhibit angiogenesis and stimulate elimination of carcinogens. These fruits, especially blueberries and bilberries (Seeram et al. 2006), also contain pigments called *anthocyanidins* and *proanthocyanidins*, which stimulate cancer-cell apoptosis. (Other sources of proanthocyanidins are cinnamon and dark chocolate.) These fruits don't cause a blood-sugar spike, so there's no excessive insulin or IGF-1 elevation. Ellagic acid, in particular, has other beneficial properties, such as detoxifying cells and blocking transformation of numerous environmental carcinogens, protecting cells from their action on the DNA (Labrecque et al. 2005). Ellagic acid also stimulates elimination of toxins from the cellular environment. Cherries contain glucaric acid, which detoxifies xenoestrogens from the body (Walaszek et al. 1998).

## CITRUS FRUITS

The familiar citrus fruits—orange, lemon, grapefruit, and tangerine—contain anti-inflammatory flavonoids. There's evidence that the flavonoids tangeretin and nobiletin, extracted from tangerine peel, penetrate cancer cells in the brain, causing apoptosis and preventing them from invading other cells (Rooprai et al. 2001). You can grate and sprinkle organic citrus fruit peel (ensure that it's organic since the peel accumulates pesticides) onto salads or even breakfast cereals.

## Pomegranate Juice

Used medicinally in Persian and other Middle Eastern cultures for centuries, pomegranate juice has well-established anti-inflammatory and antioxidant properties. Its anti-inflammatory component is apparently from blocking NF-$k$B, and it can considerably slow the growth of even the most aggressive forms of prostate cancer (Pantuck et al. 2006). NF-$k$B, as mentioned in chapter 1, plays a central role in the immune system and activates genes that control inflammation and cell growth. Daily use of pomegranate juice has cut the growth rate of established prostate cancers by two thirds. An eight-ounce glass a day is recommended (ibid.).

## Red Wine

In Europe, wine is part of many afternoon or evening meals. In the right amount, wine is a "live" food with nourishing properties. Of course, in excess it's an intoxicating drug, but what's the right amount? A French doctor might tell you three glasses a day, a German doctor two glasses, and a Danish doctor one. In the United States alcohol is widely regarded as a drug rather than a useful source of nourishment. As mentioned earlier in this chapter, the polyphenol resveratrol, found in the grape skins and therefore in much higher quantities in red wine than white, has gained wide attention for its cholesterol-lowering properties. Resveratrol can slow down cancer progression by blocking NF-$k$B (Manna, Mukhopadhyay, and Aggarwal 2000). For the cancer patient, red wine also provides stress reduction. If you don't drink very often, your sensitivity will permit you to feel relaxed by consuming a small amount, maybe less than a single glass. The hazards of misuse are obvious: if you have a genetic tendency toward alcoholism, even one drink could lead down a destructive path. A downside for anyone is that alcohol has a powerful influence on blood sugar, as diabetics know. Drinking too much can erase the potential benefits of occasional, moderate use.

## Probiotics

Probiotics are preparations containing healthful bacteria. Healthful bacteria are found naturally in "live" foods, like yogurt, sauerkraut, miso, and many kinds of pickled and preserved traditional foods. Before the days of refrigeration or nitrate preservatives for meat, forcemeats like sausages consisted of raw meat, and various herbs and spices (which are antioxidants as well as flavor enhancers), and were pushed into a casing to protect them from air and prevent harmful oxidation. Over the months, the meats "cured," allowing healthful bacteria like *Lactobacillus plantarum* to grow, turning dead meat into a live food, rich in enzymes and healthful microbes. Many natural-food stores carry good-quality yogurt, sauerkraut, miso, and even bacterial cultures in capsules or in starters for homemade live foods. In terms of general health, ensuring intake of healthful bacteria is an important factor in protecting the immune system. These bacteria can prevent colds in fatigue sufferers, who have particularly vulnerable immune systems (Cox et al. 2008). They not only improve the bowel's efficiency but also have a documented ability to prevent colon cancer (Wollowski, Rechkemmer, and Pool-Zobel 2001).

## HOW MUCH CANCER-PREVENTING FOOD DO YOU EAT?

Add the following points for cancer-preventing foods in your diet: one point for weekly use, and three points for daily use. Add three points to the total if you eat mostly organic foods, and five points if your diet is all organic:

_____ Fresh vegetables, steamed and raw

_____ Grains low on the glycemic index

_____ Olive oil, macadamia nut oil, unrefined coconut oil

_____ Meat, butter from grass-fed cows

_____ Eggs, poultry from free-range birds

_____ Almond milk, hazelnut milk, rice milk

_____ Olives

_____ Beans, hummus

_____ Multigrain bread

_____ Fruits (peeled and washed, if not organic)

_____ Tap water filtered by reverse osmosis

Subtract the following points for cancer-promoting foods in your diet: one point for weekly use, and three points for daily use:

_____ Foods high on the glycemic index

_____ Hydrogenated or partially hydrogenated oils

_____ Conventional dairy products (high in omega-6 fatty acids)

_____ Fried foods, potato chips

_____ Red meat, unless from grass-fed animals (high in omega-6 fatty acids)

_____ Eggs, poultry, unless from grass-fed animals (high in omega-6 fatty acids)

_____     Fruit and vegetable peels, if not organic

_____     Unfiltered tap water

You want a positive number here. If you scored five or below, devote some attention to changing your diet.

Not Perfect? Oh well, join the club. You don't have to be perfect to maintain health and longevity. If you're very sick, you might want to practice following a cancer-fighting diet as closely as possible for five days at a time to find out what diet works best for you. Many people find that their tastes change and that feeling good—the real goal—is addictive.

# GETTING STARTED

It takes some planning to change your dietary habits. The first step is to plan your menu for a week. Look up recipes online and in natural-food cookbooks. With a little practice, you'll soon have the skill to make vegetables taste good without adding a lot of fat or salt.

### Dietary Recommendations

> Detoxify through your diet; eat organic foods and avoid sugar, alcohol, and other stimulants.

> Avoid cancer-promoting foods and opt for cancer-fighting foods as much as possible.

> Balance your fatty-acid intake.

> Eat lightly in the evening, emphasizing carbohydrates. Eat higher protein foods in the morning and afternoon.

To prevent cancer or fight it, choose foods that:

> Boost immune-system activity: mushrooms, carotenoids (carrots and beets), seaweeds.

> Block development of new blood vessels (antiangiogenesis): green tea, cruciferous vegetables, polyphenols from fruit and red wine, flaxseeds.

> Detoxify carcinogens in our internal environment: green tea, turmeric, seaweeds, polyphenols from fruit and red wine, citrus fruits.

> Prevent and stop inflammation: omega-3 fatty acids, green tea, turmeric, ginger, pomegranate juice, flaxseeds.

> Block mechanisms that set the stage for metastasis: seaweeds, foods and supplements that block angiogenesis and support immune function.

> Induce cancer-cell apoptosis (cell death): garlic, cruciferous vegetables, turmeric, ginger, polyphenols from fruit and red wine, citrus fruits.

> Act as antioxidants: garlic, carotenoids, ginger, pomegranate juice.

> Reduce insulin and IGF-1: garlic, bilberries, burdock, fenugreek.

> Block cancer-cell development: polyphenols from fruit and red wine, omega-3 fatty acids, flaxseeds.

# CHAPTER 6

# Cancer-Fighting Supplements

This chapter covers the substantial research on the benefits of taking dietary supplements to enhance the outcome of cancer treatment and prevent its recurrence while improving quality of life (Prasad et al. 2001).

Numerous studies have focused on the use of supplements—including vitamins, minerals, plant-based antioxidants, and herbs—their effects on cancer prevention and treatment, and their compatibility with conventional cancer drugs. The great majority of evidence supports using nutritional supplementation for longer survival and for improved chemotherapy and radiation outcomes (Prasad et al. 1999). Though most oncologists don't know this area in depth, it's a growing body of knowledge. The scientific studies cited in this chapter are merely the tip of the iceberg.

## THE DIETARY SUPPLEMENTS CONTROVERSY

**Antioxidants in General:** Oncologists have been reluctant to let their patients use antioxidants for fear that it might interfere with the success of chemotherapy and radiation treatments. These treatments attempt to "oxidize" (burn out) the tumor, and they fear that antioxidants would oppose this process. One prominent cancer expert, Dr. Charles Simone, an internist, medical oncologist, tumor immunologist, and radiation oncologist who has worked with the National Cancer Institute and is a former medical school professor, has a different and unequivocal position: antioxidants and other nutrients enhance the effects of cancer treatments, decrease their side effects, and protect normal tissues, so the 900,000 cancer patients per year who receive radiation therapy and the 50,000 patients who get chemotherapy should be encouraged to use them (Simone, Simone, and Simone 1997). Dr. Simone's conclusions are based on weighing the results of 280 research studies, including research on 8,521 patients, that consistently show benefits against "a single interview in the *New York Times* in 1997 that was not based on published scientific work and a single research paper involving mouse cells" (Simone II et al. 2007), alleging that vitamin C interferes with chemotherapy and radiation. Dr. Simone further states that "antioxidants and other nutrients do not interfere with chemotherapy or radiation, but instead decrease toxicity and may improve response rates and overall survival" (ibid.).

However, oncologists routinely treat with antioxidant drugs along with chemotherapy, and there's no reported inhibition of their effect on clinical results. This is another reason the therapeutic benefits of nutritional antioxidants, which are nontoxic and from food sources, shouldn't be ignored (Moss 2000). Some such antioxidants are used very aggressively in high doses administered intravenously, which has been shown to improve outcomes (Pathak et al. 2005).

**Vitamin C:** Using vitamin C in cancer treatment was the first point of controversy over supplement use for cancer in 1997, when a front-page article in the *New York Times* quoted a spokesman from Memorial Sloan-Kettering Cancer Center, who announced that large doses of vitamin C could weaken chemotherapy's effects on cancer patients (Brody 1997). The supposed supporting research came *two years later* in the form of a mouse study that showed that there was more vitamin C in cancer cells than surrounding cells (Gottlieb 1999). That was the sole foundation for the subsequent controversy. However, another vitamin C study was published in the *Proceedings of the National Academy of Sciences* that gave the opposite message: that daily high-dose vitamin C treatment "significantly decreased growth rates" of ovarian, pancreatic, and malignant brain tumors in mice (Chen et al. 2008). Since the 1970s, numerous studies have focused on the use of vitamin C for cancer treatment (Null et al. 1997), and many human studies show that low vitamin C intake is a risk factor for cancer (Block 1991).

In 2006 Canadian doctors published clinical successes using vitamin C for cancer (Padayatty et al. 2006), but the use of vitamin C to treat cancer began in 1971 (Potter and McMichael 1986). One early study of 300 incurable cancer patients receiving 2,500 milligrams a day of vitamin C combined with surgery, radiation, and some chemotherapy showed that there was a significant survival benefit in 266 patients, particularly those with stomach, colon, and bladder cancer (Moffat, Cameron, and Campbell 1983). A 1976 study showed that intravenous vitamin C improved length and quality of life in terminal cancer patients. Doctors Ewan Cameron and Linus Pauling treated 500 terminal cancer patients who hadn't benefited from conventional treatment, and saw increased longevity and reduced pain with the vitamin C treatment (Cameron and Pauling 1976). These results were disputed by studies at the Mayo Clinic, which showed no tangible benefit from vitamin C administration (Creagan et al. 1979; Moertel et al. 1985).

Defenders of vitamin C said that the first Mayo Clinic study (Creagan et al. 1979) didn't measure blood plasma concentrations of vitamin C and were attempting to evaluate its efficacy with insufficient doses (Padayatty et al. 2004). The second study (Moertel et al. 1985) was ended abruptly after two months, and there was suspicion that the placebo group had also been using vitamin C (Block and Mead 2003). The Cameron and Pauling study (1976) had used both intravenous vitamin C, which delivers much higher serum levels of the vitamin, and the oral form, but the Mayo Clinic studies used only oral vitamin C. The Cameron and Pauling study used vitamin C as sodium ascorbate, which some nutritionists say is a more therapeutic form (Fonorow 2007). Other researchers who've studied vitamin C for cancer haven't used it separately from other vitamins (Hannes et al. 1991). Japanese doctors also showed that vitamin C significantly prolonged survival time (Murata, Morishige, and Yamaguchi 1982). Some reports also indicated that high doses of medically administered vitamin C eliminate metastases (Riordan, Jackson, and Riordan 1996). Vitamin C can also protect the body from the side effects of radiation therapy (Garcia-Alejo Hernández et al. 1989).

Almost a hundred studies since the 1970s have shown the preventive properties of vitamin C, including protection from oral, pancreatic, stomach, esophageal, cervical, breast, lung, and rectal cancers (Null et al. 1997). The way it works appears to be in its anti-inflammatory and antioxidant properties, and its ability to increase NK cell activity.

**Vitamin E:** Vitamin E is the other well-known antioxidant that has been the subject of controversy, because it was evaluated as a possible risk factor for lung cancer. You'll recall that in the Canadian study mentioned in chapter 1 (Meyer et al. 2008), researchers discovered that the group at risk from taking the vitamins was limited to the subpopulation of cigarette smokers, the people who continued smoking during radiation treatment. The key factor was that the patients who continued to smoke were the group at greater risk, but it also may be significant that the vitamins used in the Canadian study were not natural vitamins but, rather, synthetic substitutes. The research questionnaire didn't distinguish between synthetic and natural vitamins. The lesson from these studies could be that smokers should avoid synthetic antioxidants because of some interaction between them and the chemicals from tobacco smoke. This warning could probably extend to prescription antioxidants sometimes used in chemotherapy as well (Simone II et al. 2007).

Natural vitamin E is a safe and effective antioxidant for cancer prevention and treatment. Experienced nutritionists recommend using natural vitamin E, which is labeled with such names as "d-alpha-tocopherol" and "d-beta-tocopherol" (Burton et al. 1998). Synthetic vitamin E is listed as "dl-tocopherol." For the best results it's important to use a supplement that contains the full spectrum of vitamin E components: the tocopherols (alpha, beta, gamma, and delta) and the tocotrienols (alpha, beta, gamma, and delta) (Handelman et al. 1994).

Besides helping prevent cancer, vitamin E can help with some of conventional treatment's side effects. Vitamin E prevented mucositis (inflammation of the oral membranes) caused by chemotherapy, and improved treatment response rate in leukemia patients (Lopez et al. 1994). This was repeated with another group of eighteen patients receiving chemotherapy. Out of nine patients who took vitamin E, six had their mouth lesions heal, but only one out of the nine taking the placebo experienced improvement (Wadleigh et al. 1992).

Vitamin E can also prevent hair loss from chemotherapy. Sixteen patients undergoing chemotherapy with Adriamycin (doxorubicin), which usually causes hair loss, were given vitamin E daily, and eleven of them experienced no hair loss. Taking vitamin E at least three days before chemotherapy began resulted in the highest success rate (Wood 1985).

Another side effect of chemotherapy is neuropathy, which is usually experienced as a sensation of numbness, tingling, or both, often in the feet and lower legs. A study of patients taking cisplatin, paclitaxel, or both compared a group taking vitamin E to a group who didn't. Neuropathy occurred in 25 percent of the vitamin E group and 73.3 percent of the control group (Argyriou et al. 2005).

Vitamin E may also play a preventive role against prostate cancer. A study of 500 men found that the gamma-tocopherol component of vitamin E, not just alpha-tocopherol, was associated with a fivefold reduction of cancer risk (Helzlsouer et al. 2000).

A researcher at Wake Forest University (Schwenke 2002) compiled the enormous amount of data on vitamin E and concluded that vitamin E appears to play a role in preventing breast cancer. In this case, it's not the alpha-tocopherol that's effective but the gamma-tocopherol and the tocotrienols.

The most effective form of vitamin E is the mixed tocopherols that contain all of these significant factors (ibid). The recommended dosage of either gamma or mixed tocopherols is up to 1,000 milligrams per day, taken with food (European Food Safety Authority 2008).

**Beta-Carotene:** As mentioned earlier, beta-carotene (or provitamin A) is the pigment in carrots and other yellow and orange vegetables. It metabolizes into vitamin A, which the liver uses for numerous functions. Dietary beta-carotene is a possible cancer preventive. One controversial study (Omenn et al. 1994) found that beta-carotene supplementation increased the risk for lung cancer; large doses of synthetic beta-carotene were used in this study. Not only is the synthetic form questionable, but also in the synthetic form, beta-carotene is separated from other beneficial carotenes that need to work together. This study, like the discredited Montreal study (Bairati et al. 2005), showed negative findings that pertained to a group that continued to smoke tobacco during treatment with synthetic vitamin C.

This is further evidence that there's an important difference between synthetic and food-based beta-carotene supplements. High doses of food beta-carotenes, such as in carrot juice or beet juice, are perfectly safe and helpful. Some natural cancer therapies recommend several fresh carrot-based vegetable juices a day (Ferrell 1998).

# SYNTHETIC VS. FOOD-DERIVED VITAMINS

There's an important distinction in quality between synthetic and natural, food-derived vitamins. Cheap synthetic supplements, called "isolates," have a lower efficiency and sometimes no effect at all compared to natural vitamins. While this issue remains controversial for many vitamins, even critics of supplementation agree that it's necessary to have vitamin E in a complete, natural form. If your goal is to prevent or treat cancer, high-quality supplements are essential. If the vitamin product is natural and food derived, its label should say so, and also declare that the product is free of unsafe additives or allergens, as well as convey the extent of its quality-control procedures. Standard quality-control certifications are in place for vitamin and mineral products. Look for a product that's produced at an ISO- or NSF-certified facility. An ISO rating shows that the manufacturer has followed a set of quality standards to be certified, but the highest rating is the NSF Good Manufacturing Processes (GMP) certification.

# RECOMMENDED SUPPLEMENTS

A number of supplements have been tested for use with conventional cancer treatment. Following are several that you can use to improve treatment outcome, help maintain quality of life, or both, as well as reduce side effects and enhance well-being.

## AHCC

AHCC is a cultured mushroom product used in over 700 clinics and hospitals in Japan to protect the immune system and reduce side effects in cancer patients receiving chemotherapy and radiation (Kenner 2001). Many people in Japan take it to prevent cancer and maintain general health. AHCC has been researched in Japan, China, the United States, and Thailand (International AHCC Research Association 2006), and results show that it works both to prevent and treat numerous diseases. AHCC improves the immune system's ability to recognize tumors (Gao et al. 2006), increases the activity of immune "scavenger cells" (NK cells) (Ghoneum et al. 1995), extends life span in advanced stages of cancer (Matsui et al. 2002), and improves five-year survival rates even in advanced stages (Kawaguchi 2003; Cowawintaweewat et al. 2006). AHCC strengthens the effects of chemotherapy, protects the immune system from its side effects, and prevents metastasis (Hirose et al. 2007). The recommended dosage of AHCC for cancer patients six weeks ahead of and during chemotherapy is 3 to 6 grams, three times a day (Cowawintaweewat et al. 2006).

## Astragalus

An herb used for centuries in Chinese medicine, astragalus has been well researched and is regarded as one of the most powerful immune system boosters. It has been used in China since the 1970s to protect the immune system from the side effects of cancer chemotherapy (Sun, Chang, and Yu 1981). Among its many immune system enhancements are its ability to stimulate white cell activity, including NK cells, and to increase production of the antitumor cytokines interferon and tumor necrosis factor (Wei et al. 2003). Astragalus actually strengthens the effect of platinum-based chemotherapy in advanced non-small-cell lung cancer (McCulloch et al. 2006b). Astragalus is usually taken in doses of 9 to 15 grams a day of the dried root, 750 to 1,500 milligrams of the powdered extract, or 2 to 6 milliliters a day of the 5-to-1 tincture (Wassef 1998).

## Avemar

Avemar is a biologically active, cultured wheat-germ extract developed in Hungary for medical use. Animal, cell-line, and human-clinical studies support its use as a medication, particularly to complement conventional cancer therapy (Boros, Nichelatti, and Shoenfeld 2005). Avemar has been shown to have a significantly therapeutic effect in controlled human trials in treating primary colorectal cancer (Jakab et al. 2003), stage III melanoma (Demidov et al. 2002), and stages III and IV oral cancer (Barabás and Németh 2006). Avemar consistently enhances quality of life and reduces chemotherapy side effects, as well as prevents chemotherapy-induced suppression of immune function. Avemar also significantly reduced the risk of febrile neutropenia (decrease in white blood cells that often leads to infection) in children receiving chemotherapy for leukemia (Garami et al. 2004). Another study showed that Avemar significantly enhanced the effect of tamoxifen on estrogen-positive breast cancer cells (Marcsek et al. 2004). The dose for adults is one packet (9 grams) twice a day, and for children, one packet is divided into two doses (Jakab et al. 2003).

## Coenzyme $Q_{10}$

Found in every cell of the body, *coenzyme $Q_{10}$*, also called $CoQ_{10}$, is a vital nutrient that's instrumental in cells' conversion of fuel into energy. It was developed as a nutritional supplement in Japan fifty years ago, where it has since been used as a prescription drug for cardiovascular and brain health. Safe even at very high doses, it has been studied for its therapeutic and protective effects in cancer treatment since the 1990s. Because of its powerful tissue-protecting properties, medical researchers decided to study its potential for preventing chemotherapy-related tissue damage (Combs et al. 1977), and eventually research progressed to human studies.

Doctors at the University of Texas Institute for Biomedical Research found data on improved survival rates in humans and "striking" responses to therapy in patients with lung, colon, and prostate cancer as well as other conditions (Folkers et al. 1993). Danish doctors carried out a study using $CoQ_{10}$ with thirty-two high-risk, advanced breast-cancer patients. Though all of the women had had surgery, residual tumor mass remained. They were given vitamins C and E with selenium, essential fatty acids, and 90 milligrams a day of $CoQ_{10}$. Six of the thirty-two women showed partial tumor regression; that is, not only did the tumors stop growing, but they also got smaller. None of the women showed metastases, and all reported improved quality of life (Lockwood et al. 1994). The dose was raised to 390 milligrams a day for two of the women, and within three months, there was no residual tumor tissue and they were in "excellent condition" (Lockwood, Moesgaard, and Folkers 1994). Dr. Knud Lockwood, the lead researcher in the study, indicated that he had never before seen a spontaneous complete regression of a 1.5 to 2 centimeter breast tumor or a comparable regression in any conventional antitumor therapy (ibid.). In 2007 researchers in Madras, India, studied eighty-four breast-cancer chemotherapy patients who were primarily taking tamoxifen, along with $CoQ_{10}$, niacin, and riboflavin (two B vitamins). From analyzing tumor markers in the blood, the researchers concluded that $CoQ_{10}$ "reduces … the risk of cancer recurrence and metastases" (Premkumar et al. 2007). (A newer form of $CoQ_{10}$, called ubiquinol, claims to be even more effective because it's absorbed more efficiently (Hosoe et al. 2007). The women who experienced remission were using almost 400 milligrams a day. A typical dose for daily use is 30 to 60 milligrams a day. To protect the heart from chemotherapy side effects, use 100 to 200 milligrams a day (Iarussi et al. 1994).

## Folate

Part of the vitamin B complex, folate has attracted attention as a preventive for cervical and colon cancers. In one study, HPV (human papillomavirus) infection did not lead to cervical dysplasia (abnormal, sometimes precancerous cells) in women with high levels of folate in the blood (Piyathilake et al. 2007). Folate also prevents ovarian cancer (Larsson, Giovannucci, and Wolk 2004). Having adequate levels of folate in the blood prevents colon cancer. Colon cancer risk was 60 percent less in men who took at least 239 micrograms of folate a day, compared to men who took less than 103.3 micrograms a day (Su and Arab 2001). Women who'd taken over 400 micrograms a day for fifteen years had a 75 percent reduced risk of colon cancer (Giovannucci et al. 1998b). Because folic acid is the synthetic version of folate, opt for folate when shopping for this important nutrient.

## Ginseng

Besides showing both cancer-fighting (Lee et al. 1997) and cancer-preventive activity (Yun, Choi, and Yun 2001), ginseng can also help the more than 90 percent of cancer patients who suffer from extreme lethargy and low energy levels before, during, or after treatment. Sixty-two percent of cancer patients undergoing chemotherapy or radiation treatment felt relief from fatigue after taking between 750 and 2,000 milligrams of powdered American ginseng, according to cancer experts at the forty-third annual meeting of the American Society of Clinical Oncology in Chicago in 2007 (Barton et al. 2007).

## Minerals

**Iodine:** Found in many foods but especially abundant in seafood, iodine may help prevent cancer, particularly breast cancer. Iodine tests now evaluate women's breast-cancer susceptibility. Though you can supplement iodine with kelp and other sea products, it's better to consult with a health care provider before using a pure iodine supplement, such as Lugol's solution (Funahashi et al. 1996).

**Magnesium:** Another important mineral to supplement, magnesium is depleted by excess sugar and alcohol, and deficiency is very common. Magnesium is important for many vital functions, including its role as a well-known bone-hardness factor, and research also points to cancer protection as another of its roles. In the case of tumors, high magnesium levels prevent carcinogenesis (Durlach et al. 1986). The orotate or aspartate form of magnesium can be taken in higher doses. A recommended daily dose is around 500 to 1,000 milligrams when headache, muscle spasm, or high sugar or alcohol consumption is present. Doses as high as 4,500 milligrams have been used for headache pain in children and adolescents (Grazzi et al. 2005). Increase the dose to 1,500 to 2,000 milligrams for pain or tension from alcohol or sugar overconsumption.

**Selenium:** Playing an important role in immunity, selenium is necessary for proper functioning of the white blood cells that protect us from infections, and it's also necessary in order for vitamin E to properly play its role (Arthur, McKenzie, and Beckett 2003). Test animals with cancer survived significantly longer when given high doses of vitamin E, selenium, and vitamin C. Complete tumor remission occurred in 16.8 percent of the animals (Evangelou et al. 1997). High selenium levels in the blood protect against prostate cancer. According to a Stanford University study, men with adequate selenium have a fivefold decrease in prostate-cancer risk (Brooks et al. 2001). Grains, beans, meat, and fish are good sources of selenium, but since selenium levels decline with age (and prostate cancer risk increases with age), supplementation should be considered for the elderly. Dosage is 200 micrograms a day for cancer prevention (Clark et al. 1996).

**Zinc:** A mineral that catalyzes many types of biochemical reactions, zinc also affects immunity, because low zinc levels result in low NK cell activity (Prasad 1998). Patients with digestive-tract cancers who were receiving chemotherapy were randomly assigned doses of supplemental zinc and selenium. All of the patients were malnourished, but 70 percent of the group receiving the mineral supplements had no further deterioration of nutritional status, more energy, and a better appetite. In the control group, only 20 percent experienced no further nutritional impairment (Federico et al. 2001). Sources of zinc in the diet include many types of seafood, especially oysters, meat, yogurt, and cheese. Vegetarian sources high in zinc are beans, cashews, and almonds. Daily recommended dietary intake for healthy people is 11 milligrams for adult men and 8 milligrams for women (Institute of Medicine 2002).

## Proteolytic Enzymes

Proteolytic enzymes digest proteins, and they're useful not only for their anti-inflammatory ability (Ito et al. 1979) but also for tumor reduction (Leipner and Saller 2000). They can also break down proteins that damage the kidneys, as well as break through a tumor's protective shell and expose it to immune surveillance. In a study of 166 stage III multiple myeloma (bone-marrow cancer) patients, lives were extended in a group taking a daily dose of proteolytic enzymes. The treated group survived eighty-three months, compared to forty-seven months in the untreated group (Sakalová et al. 2001). Proteolytic enzymes can also protect from some of the collateral damage of radiation therapy and prevent damage to mucous membranes, skin, the digestive tract, and the bladder (Dale et al. 2001). Bromelain (pineapple enzyme), papain (papaya enzyme), and pancreatin (pancreatic extract, usually from sheep or pig) are the three enzymes most frequently used in combinations, and are safe and well tested.

## Vitamin D

Vitamin D can prevent colorectal cancer, according to research published in the *American Journal of Preventive Medicine*. A meta-analysis (an analysis of other research reports) on vitamin D and cancer susceptibility showed that the highest serum levels of vitamin D reduced the risk of colorectal cancer by 50 percent. To achieve these levels, it's necessary to take at least 1,000 to 2,000 IU per day (Gorham et al. 2007). Women taking higher doses of vitamin D and calcium have a lower risk of developing breast cancer, according to another study (Lin et al. 2007). In addition to being anti-inflammatory, vitamin D inhibits the growth of new blood vessels (Kalkunte et al. 2005). According to a fairly recent study, 2,000 IU per day of vitamin D and moderate sun exposure can reduce breast-cancer risk by 50 percent (Garland et al. 2007).

William Grant, former senior research scientist at NASA, Langley, and director of the Sunlight, Nutrition, and Health Research Center in San Francisco, indicates that there are over hundreds of peer-reviewed scientific studies supporting the use of vitamin D for cancer treatment and prevention (Grant 2004). The preferred form of vitamin D is vitamin D3, and the daily dosage should be at least 1,000 IU (Grant and Holick 2005).

*Supplemental Energy Boost*

M. R., aged 58, was treated for prostate cancer with radioactive seed implants. Though he was in charge of a large construction project, he began to feel so tired that he thought he'd have to take time off. He didn't follow a special diet but used supplements prescribed by his acupuncturist, including a mushroom extract, an antioxidant supplement, and whey protein powder. Besides regaining his energy, which enabled him to face his heavy workload, he experienced the cessation of what had been an uncomfortable rectal burning. Thus his response to complementary treatment with supplements was successful.

# DISCUSSING SUPPLEMENTS WITH YOUR ONCOLOGIST

The medical environment is intimidating enough as it is, in part because of all the choices you have to make, but even more so if you have to make choices that your medical consultants or family might oppose. In these cases, use a consultant who's an expert on nutrition and dietary supplements. If there's insufficient evidence to use an antioxidant but you feel that it would benefit you, you may choose to discuss with your health care practitioner whether it would be possible to schedule its use in a way that avoids conflict or interference with your treatment. If it's necessary to avoid a certain antioxidant or supplement during chemotherapy because your oncologist isn't comfortable with it, you can find out the half-life of the drugs, which is usually fewer than seventy-two hours. Most antioxidants stay in the blood for about twenty-four hours, with the exception of oil-soluble substances, such as vitamins A and E, and others, which can stay in the blood for several days. You can use the antioxidants after the half-life of the chemotherapy drugs.

## DO YOU NEED SUPPLEMENTS?

While not everyone needs to take supplements to be healthy, some people find that they feel much better when taking appropriate supplements, especially during or between treatments. Here's a questionnaire that should get you thinking about some areas where supplementation might be useful. Circle "Y" for yes or "N" for no:

Y or N _____ Do you take supplements?

Y or N _____ Do you know a knowledgeable health care provider who can help you choose the right supplements? Do you take supplements based on recommendations from a health care professional?

Y or N _____ Do you feel that you have enough energy?

Y or N _____ Do you get tired easily?

Y or N _____ Do you catch cold easily?

Y or N _____ If you catch cold, does it persist for two weeks or more?

Y or N _____ Does a cold move into your chest quickly?

Y or N _____ Do you have swollen glands in your neck?

Y or N  _____  Do you have frequent infections?

Y or N  _____  Do you have a chronic cough?

Y or N  _____  Do you feel that your sex drive is low?

Low immunity and fatigue may indicate a need for more than what we can get from food in the short term, so you may want to consider adding supplements. Professional advice to target your needs will save you money in the long run.

Many of the supplements in this chapter are simply foods. For example, AHCC is fermented mushrooms, and Avemar is simply fermented wheat germ. Proteolytic enzymes are made from such sources as tropical fruits and animal tissues. You learned in the previous chapter that many foods have therapeutic properties, including turmeric, garlic, ginger, and others. Using supplements is no different from having yogurt, sauerkraut, or miso in the diet except that they're in capsules or packets. Since there's no clear line between food and supplement in these cases, it's unlikely to be inappropriate. Vitamins and minerals are also safe to take, provided guidelines are followed. If you're undergoing cancer treatment, work closely with a nutrition-oriented health care provider if you intend to take high doses. If you're undergoing chemotherapy and radiation, check for contraindications between the drugs you're taking and the supplements. While contraindications are few, it's important to know if they exist.

# CHAPTER 7

# Lifestyle and Risk Factors

Because of improved hygiene and modern medicine, today people live longer but when they die, it's most often of old-age diseases, such as cancer (Miniño et al. 2007). In an older population a higher cancer rate is to be expected, but we still need to heed warnings about our harmful modern lifestyle and environmental degradation. The increase of cancer since the 1940s in industrialized nations accelerated after 1975, especially among *young people*. The cancer rate in women under age forty-five grew 1.6 percent a year between 1975 and 1994, and 1.8 percent in men (Ries et al. 2002), which can't be explained by the aging population theory. Nor can it explain the massive increase in the cancer rate in children and adolescents, especially since 1970 (Steliarova-Foucher et al. 2004). The argument that earlier detection has increased cancer statistics also falls short, because there's also an increase in the rates of cancers that aren't easily detectable by screening, such as lung, pancreatic, and brain cancers, and lymphoma (Ries et al. 2002).

Even though we all produce microscopic malignant cells, they grow into tumors five to fifty times more frequently in the West than in East Asia, especially breast, colon, and prostate cancers (Stewart and Kleihues 2003). Even in modern, industrialized Japan, cancer development occurs at a significantly lower rate. In Japanese men who died of causes other than cancer, autopsies showed that there were just as many precancerous microscopic tumors as in Western men (Yatani et al. 1988), which seems to indicate that something in the Japanese lifestyle prevented these tumors from developing any further. In Japanese men living in the West, the cancer rate approaches that of the West within a generation or two (Boyle and Levin 2008). Something in the Western lifestyle interferes with our bodies' ability to defend against these abnormal growths.

How can we protect ourselves against the environmental degradation and food-production industrialization that has taken place since the 1940s?

# LIFESTYLE FACTORS

**Diet:** When I lived in Japan I discovered that the Japanese diet is recognized as one of the healthiest in the world. I knew that the average life span of the Japanese was around five years longer than that of Americans. In my clinical work I saw many men in states of partial undress, and was amazed to see men in their seventies with firm skin and supple muscles. Their diet was the only explanation I could come up with. Osaka was crowded with people and dense with noise, pollution, and electromagnetic fields, and people seemed rushed and busy. But every day, people ate "live" foods filled with healthful bacteria, such as miso and Japanese pickles. Rice and vegetables were prominent, along with small amounts of meat, usually fish, and green tea was ever present. I myself thrived on this diet and began to appreciate feeling a sense of nourishment and well-being after a meal instead of feeling tired and still vaguely hungry. Further, you seldom see overweight people in Japan. Obesity is another significant risk factor for cancer. This fact received recent attention in 2007 and 2008, even though the research has been recognized since at least 2001 (Bergström et al. 2001). A recent study analyzed 221 previous studies of over 250,000 cases of 20 different types of cancer, and found that the risk from obesity increases even for less common types of cancer, like leukemia (Renehan et al. 2008).

**Dental Hygiene:** A link exists between periodontal disease and the health of the rest of your body. Bacteria living in the gums and periodontal pockets are known to play a role in cardiovascular health. In 2007, Harvard School of Public Health published a study in the *Journal of the National Cancer Institute* that links periodontal disease with increased risk of pancreatic cancer. Apparently some of the bacteria in the mouth where periodontal disease is present produce carcinogenic substances (Michaud et al. 2007).

Root canals can be a risk factor in cases of constant low-grade inflammation. Tissue around the dead teeth and their bone sockets is sometimes inflamed, which can drain immune resources. As you've learned, inflammation is an important promoter of cancer. Integrative cancer clinics in Europe often pay close attention to the condition of the teeth with regard to these focal infections when treating cancer or other chronic diseases.

**Exercise:** Research shows that it doesn't necessarily take strenuous exercise to get the benefit and prevention value of exercise. Walk every day, and take a long walk a few times a week. Take an exercise break on your lunch hour, walk or bike as much as you can, and go dancing (Patel et al. 2003).

**Sunshine and Natural Light:** Vitamin D deficiency is common in breast cancer diagnosis, and women diagnosed with breast cancer who are low in vitamin D are twice as likely to have metastasis as those with sufficient vitamin D (Goodwin et al. 2008). Thus vitamin D supplementation may be necessary. At more northern latitudes, some research suggests that exposure to UVB rays may not be adequate during the months between late fall and early spring to meet our basic need for vitamin D (Webb, Kline, and Holick 1988). Women with sufficient sun exposure have half the risk of breast cancer, according to a Stanford University study of 4,000 women (John et al. 2007). A previous study also showed a reduced risk of prostate cancer with higher sun exposure (John et al. 2005).

But shouldn't we avoid sunlight to prevent skin cancer? Not necessarily. Malignant melanoma occurs more frequently in places that get very little sunlight; for example, it occurs ten times as often on the islands north of Scotland as those in the Mediterranean Sea. It also frequently appears in places on the body that aren't exposed to the sun. In Scotland there are five times as many melanoma lesions on the feet as on the hands, and in Japan, 40 percent of melanomas are on the soles of the feet (Karnauchow 1995). We might be better advised to avoid too much artificial light. A Harvard researcher proposed that low levels of the hormone melatonin, which is insufficiently produced in people exposed to light at night, is responsible for a higher risk of breast cancer (Schernhammer et al. 2008). Melatonin protects from cancer, and research showed that night-shift workers have lower melatonin levels and increased risk of breast and colorectal cancers (Schernhammer et al. 2001; Schernhammer et al. 2003).

**Sufficient Sleep:** The benefits of sleep, both for cancer prevention and recovery, are now established. Sleep in the dark, because the slightest bit of light can disrupt sleep hormones and neurotransmitters, such as melatonin and serotonin; get to bed early, because it's especially beneficial to be asleep during the hours between 11:00 p.m. and 3:00 a.m. (Zhdanova and Wurtman 1997); avoid TV or computer use near bedtime; don't have snacks, especially sweets, near bedtime; and wear socks, because doing so reduces night awakenings (Sephton and Spiegel 2003). Keep your cell phone away from your bed and preferably turned off; cell phone radiation has also been linked to insomnia (Arnetz et al. 2007). A study conducted by National Cancer Institute researchers showed that not only does exercise prevent cancer and encourage sleep, but also women who sleep at least seven hours a night have a 47 percent reduced risk of breast cancer (McClain et al. 2008).

# RISK FACTORS

**Inherited Risk:** There's no doubt that we all acquire certain tendencies from our genetic heritage, which can include tendencies toward certain types of cancer. Inheriting genes that predispose you to get cancer, however, is not a death sentence. The genetic inheritance expresses itself according the body's internal environment, which we acquire through our life experience.

We often hear that someday innovations in genetic science will finally offer a cure for cancer. While it's certainly possible that genetic science will present significant medical breakthroughs, ample evidence shows that environment plays a primary role in cancer incidence. If cancer were transmitted genetically, then adopted children would have the same cancer rate as their *biological* parents, *not* their adoptive parents. However, a Danish study published in the *New*

*England Journal of Medicine* showed just the opposite (Sørensen et al. 1988), which is surprising since adoptive parents contribute no genes, only lifestyle habits. A Swedish study showed that genetically identical twins don't share the same cancer risk but that lifestyle habits are the main source of risk for the disease (ibid.). Another example is the study that showed that women with high-risk BRCA genes had a much higher breast-cancer incidence by age fifty before World War II, compared to after (King, Marks, and Mandell 2003). Breast-cancer risk was 24 percent in women born before 1940, but 67 percent in women born since then. The study also pointed out that weight control and physical exercise played a significant role in delayed onset. Recent evidence also highlights the fact that healthy living can switch off the activity of genes that promote cancer development (Ornish et al. 2008).

**Potential Risks from Drugs:** Be sure to tell each doctor you consult about any drugs you're taking that were prescribed by other doctors. In my experience, all too often doctors don't know what their patients are taking. Some drugs are potential risk factors for cancer or its recurrence. A well-known example is the breast-cancer drug tamoxifen, which has been found to increase uterine-cancer risk. This raises concerns for women who are taking it for breast-cancer prevention (Bergman et al. 2000). Certain types of antidepressants, such as the tricyclic ones, for example, Elavil (amitriptyline) and Norpramin (desipramine), can also increase cancer risk (Cotterchio et al. 2000), and there's also a potential cancer risk for women using fertility drugs to become pregnant (Calderon-Margalit et al. 2009). On the other hand, some drugs, such as some of the statins and anti-inflammatory drugs like ibuprofen and even aspirin, can have preventive effects (Nelson and Harris 2000), but all of these drugs have risks and side effects, and therefore shouldn't be used alone to prevent cancer. The drug danazol, a synthetic form of the hormone progesterone used to treat endometriosis, can increase the risk of ovarian cancer (Cottreau et al. 2003).

Hormone replacement therapy (HRT) is another risk factor. Findings by the Women's Health Initiative show that women who took estrogen and progestin pills for as little as a couple of years had a greater chance of getting cancer. When they stopped taking the hormones, the odds improved quickly, returning to a normal risk level roughly two years after quitting (Rossouw et al. 2002).

**Electromagnetic Stress:** While there's a lot of different ways to get electromagnetic stress, cell phones are now an omnipresent factor. Research from Sweden, where cell phones have been in widespread use for longer than almost anywhere, indicates that cell phones may present a potential risk hazard for brain cancer and benign tumors of the acoustic nerve (Kundi et al. 2004). A study at Tel Aviv University in Israel identifies mouth cancer as another potential danger (Sadetzki et al. 2008).

**Ionizing Radiation:** For most of us, *ionizing radiation exposure*, radiation that changes the electric charge of substances through which it passes, comes from medical and dental X-rays. Always ascertain whether X-rays are absolutely necessary to diagnose and evaluate your condition. Even before radiation's well-known hazards were studied in atomic bomb victims, as early as 1943, Manhattan Project atomic scientists Robert Oppenheimer, Enrico Fermi, and Edward Teller knew that even if the bomb didn't work, they could use the radiation as a biological weapon, for example, by poisoning the German food supply (Rhodes 1986). Another modern radiation threat is nuclear power plants. Since 1988, a few years after the accidental release of radiation at Three Mile Island Nuclear Generating Station, epidemiologists in the United States and Europe have correlated high rates of childhood cancers, especially leukemia, with living in the vicinity of a nuclear reactor (Morris and Knorr 1996).

**Tobacco Smoke:** There's immediate benefit in quitting smoking: if you quit before age fifty, you're half as likely to die of cancer over the next fifteen years (Office of the Surgeon General 1990). Nearly 40 percent of children in the United States are exposed to secondhand tobacco smoke (American Academy of Pediatrics 2009), which has been the dominant issue in recent years. What about those who are involuntarily exposed to smoke? What's their risk level? The Environmental Protection Agency considers secondhand smoke to be a risk factor for cancer. Living with a smoker increases the likelihood of developing lung cancer 20 to 30 percent, and research suggests there's an increased risk of developing other types of cancer as well (U.S. Environmental Protection Agency 1993). Lung-cancer risk is lower among both smokers and nonsmokers who eat at least five servings of vegetables and fruits a day (LeMarchand et al. 2000). Healthful eating, however, won't compensate for the ill effects of tobacco smoking. Because food-derived vitamin E and beta-carotene supplements are safe, it's recommended to get these nutrients from food as much as possible.

**Toxins from Chemicals:** Though I list chemical-toxin exposure last, it's not least in importance. Environmental chemicals are a risk factor for not only cancer but also many other diseases. Such toxins oxidize our DNA and cause genetic damage, and we know that oxidative stress is a cause of cancer. Other chemicals are not only toxic but also have hormone-like effects that can disrupt the body's metabolism, and many of the chemicals are xenoestrogens, which behave like estrogens. Laboratory scientists observed that breast cancer cells grew rapidly when stored in plastic bags, just as if they had been exposed to estrogen. Estrogen is dangerous for any kind of cancer, but the estrogen-like chemicals appear to disrupt reproductive and thyroid hormones in particular (Fernandez et al. 2008). The U.S. Environmental Protection Agency says that 100 percent of us have stored PCBs, dioxins, dichlorobenzene, and xylene in our fat tissue (Centers for Disease Control and Prevention 2005). Among the most toxic substances known, PCBs and dioxins (Carpenter 2005) are found everywhere: in the oceans, the polar ice caps, in the breast milk of Inuit women living in remote polar regions (Muckle et al. 2001), and in remote areas of the Great Lakes (U.S. Environmental Protection Agency 1998). In 1986, Public Data Access, Inc., published *Quality of Life in American Neighborhoods: Levels of Affluence, Toxic Waste, and Cancer Mortality in Residential Zip Code Areas* (Westview Press), which cites EPA data and can tell you what environmental toxins have been found near your residence.

The following table lists some of these chemicals.

## CHEMICAL TOXINS IN OUR ENVIRONMENT

Compiled from data collected from the Agency for Toxic Substances and Disease Registry of the U.S. Department of Health and Human Services, www.atsdr.cdc.gov/substances/index.asp

| Toxin | Harmful Effects | Where It's Found |
|---|---|---|
| PCBs (polychlorinated biphenyls) | Carcinogenic, teratogenic | Plastics, building materials, caulking, lubricating fluids, petroleum combustion, pesticides, inks |
| Dioxins | Carcinogenic, damaging to the liver, estrogen-like (an infamous dioxin is Agent Orange, used as a defoliant in the Vietnam War) | Plastics, pesticides |
| Styrene | Carcinogenic; releases benzene, known to cause leukemia | Styrofoam |
| Atrazine | Causes prostate hypertrophy; may cause prostate cancer | Weed killer |
| BPA (bisphenol A) | Estrogen-like, causes damage to breast and prostate | Plastic food and drink containers, food wraps, linings of metal cans, lids of mason jars |
| Phthalates | Estrogen-like, carcinogenic, lower sperm count | Vinyl shower curtains, plastic toys, plastic bottles, cosmetics and perfumes |
| Polyvinyl chloride (PVC) | Estrogen-like | Shower curtains, wires, cables, appliances, upholstery, aerosol propellants |
| Organochlorines (DDT, chlordane, lindane) | Estrogen-like, damage nerves | Pesticides; lindane is used in formulations for children's head lice |

| PBDEs (polybrominated diphenyl ethers) | Carcinogenic, neurotoxic | Flame retardants, furniture foam, polyurethane foam, textiles, consumer electronics product plastic casings, wires |
|---|---|---|
| Trichloroethylenes (TCE) | Carcinogenic | Dry cleaning, carpeting, cardboard, other manufacturing |

Shower curtains and carpets can actually release hundreds of other toxic chemicals, including benzene, methylbenzene, toluene, xylene, and formaldehyde. Formaldehyde is also found in plywood, pressed wood (bookcases, dresser drawers), and insulation.

**Toxic Metals:** Toxic metals include mercury, arsenic, lead, cadmium, nickel, and aluminum. These metals form chemical bonds with normal proteins and peptides (peptides are smaller units that form proteins; many hormones are peptides), which can trigger immune system reactions and then become new substances that aren't recognized by the immune system. Some heavy metals, such as cadmium and arsenic, are known carcinogens, but any immune system reaction can cause unresolved inflammation, which, as we know, promotes cancer (Fournié et al. 2002).

Here are some common sources of toxic metal exposure:

> Aluminum: Cooking utensils, baking powder, deodorants

> Arsenic: Seafood from coastal waters, building materials, insecticides, tobacco, paints, fossil fuel combustion

> Cadmium: Paint, dental materials, seafood, tobacco, automobile exhaust, tires, plastics, batteries, PVC pipes (cadmium is used to induce prostate cancer in test animals)

> Lead: Paint, water pipes, pottery, lead crystal, cosmetics, hair dye, metal polish, pesticides, and insecticides

> Mercury: Dental amalgam, seafood, pesticides, insecticides, various industries

There's no way to live in a cocoon and be perfectly safe. While it's impossible to avoid all of these chemicals, there are a few obvious things we can do to minimize exposure. Here are a few major, common sources of chemicals in the living environment and some alternative choices we can make:

**Strategies for Self-Care**
Cosmetics, nail polish, hair dyes and sprays, shampoo, lotions, and other skin care products: Look for natural and organic products, and avoid parabens and phthalates. Some cosmetics have

aluminum bases; some dandruff shampoos contain selenium, which is a nutritional supplement in very small amounts (measured in micrograms, or millionths of a gram); and some antiperspirants contain aluminum.

> Costume jewelry can be a source of nickel exposure.

> Dry cleaning uses triethylenes: Hang clothes out to let them "off-gas" for several hours, preferably outside, before putting them back in your closet.

> Shower curtains (PVC) release hundreds of toxic chemicals: Ventilate as much as possible or replace with other material or, ideally, a glass door.

> Shower: Since there's a much higher chlorine exposure from the shower (Brown, Bishop, and Rowan 1984), use a shower filter. If you filter your drinking and cooking water, not filtering the shower misses an important piece.

## Food and Drink Precautions

> Plastic: Avoid storing food and drink in plastic whenever possible. Use glass or porcelain instead. At the very least, don't let hot items come into contact with plastic; the same goes for styrofoam.

> Lead crystal: Lead leaches out into liquids, even after a few minutes, especially with alcohol (Guadagnino 1998).

> Tobacco smoke is a source of heavy metals, especially cadmium and arsenic, and other chemicals besides nicotine are also present.

> Baking powder often contains aluminum, but health food stores often offer some that don't.

> Hydrogenated oils (trans fats) are hazardous enough, but they also have nickel residues. Nickel is used as a catalyst to make liquid oils congeal.

> Cookware: Use glass, cast iron, carbon steel, or titanium. Aluminum and Teflon are known for their toxic hazards. Stainless steel pots can leach nickel into their contents (International Programme on Chemical Safety 1991).

> Thermoses: Avoid stainless steel and plastic thermoses; the glass-lined ones are best.

> Metal polish: Many of them contain lead.

## Things Around the House

> Household cleaning products: Use environmentally healthful liquid detergents and laundry soaps, such as are found in health food stores and specialty stores.

> Batteries contain cadmium; carefully dispose of leaking batteries. Nickel-cadmium batteries are usually recyclable.

> Paints contain cadmium and lead, especially old paints.

> Carpets: It can take months for new carpets laden with toxic chemicals to off-gas. If you have a choice, nontoxic alternatives are available; otherwise good ventilation can speed up the process of clearing out chemicals.

> Building materials are full of PVCs and other chemicals, and treated wood sometimes contains arsenates. Do not burn building materials.

> PVC pipes: Both lead and PVC pipes are highly toxic (Creech and Johnson 1974). (There are lots of lead pipes still in use across the United States.)

### House and Yard

> Insecticides, herbicides, and pesticides: A common source of heavy metals, like lead and arsenic, these substances are toxic. Public parks, and especially golf courses, are major sources of exposure, especially when they're being watered. Neighbors' lawns are also a major source of these toxins, which can get on your carpet and stay there if you wear shoes inside your house that came into contact with them.

### Health Care

> Dental amalgam fillings contain mercury and other metals. More dentists are now using composites; opt for them if possible.

---

# ASSESS YOUR EXPOSURE TO TOXINS

While there's no way to avoid all of the chemicals we're exposed to every day, there are a few things we can do. These questions will help you assess your toxic chemical exposure. Circle "Y" for yes or "N" for no, and mark in the number of points indicated for each question:

Y or N _____ Do you use tobacco? If so, every day or occasionally (every day = five points; occasionally = three points)?

Y or N _____ Are you exposed to hazardous chemicals or radiation at work (if so, add three points)?

Y or N _____ Do you have dental metals in your mouth (if so, add three points)?

These questions pertain to toxic exposures in your home (1 point for each):

Y or N    _____     Do you use aluminum cookware?

Y or N    _____     Do you use worn Teflon cookware?

Y or N    _____     Do you have lead paint or pipes in your home?

Y or N    _____     Do you use vinyl shower curtains?

Y or N    _____     Do you live near commercial agriculture fields?

Y or N    _____     Do you use skin care, hygiene, or cosmetic products containing phthalates or parabens on a daily basis?

Y or N    _____     Was your home recently constructed, or was new carpet installed recently?

We're limited in what we can do to avoid environmental toxins. A combination of diet, certain supplements, and exercise can help detoxify your body of environmental chemicals, but if your total score exceeds nine, seriously consider sauna therapy as well.

# CHAPTER 8

# Exercise

Exercising is not only for maintaining our health; it's one of many ways we can nurture ourselves. Some people have a "tough love" approach and regularly try to push the body to new limits, while others take a casual approach and just try to have fun. We've all heard that the combination of diet and exercise is a pathway to health and well-being, but there's convincing evidence that exercise is a key factor in longevity and quality of life for cancer patients.

## THE IMPACT OF EXERCISE ON THE FACTORS THAT PROMOTE CANCER GROWTH

The evidence highlights what are now likely familiar themes to you. Exercise strengthens the immune system, including NK cell activity (LaPerriere et al. 1990), reduces inflammation (Ford 2002), and lowers insulin and IGF levels (Leung et al. 2004). It also lowers excess levels of hormones such as estrogen and testosterone, which can fuel tumor growth (Friedenreich and Orenstein 2002). Exercise increases levels of pleasure neurotransmitters, like endorphins, and reduces levels of stress-related hormones, like cortisol. Thus it's useful for depression, a common symptom of chronic stress or PTSD (Woolery et al. 2004). Researchers who compared exercise to a pharmaceutical antidepressant for patients with major depression found exercise to be equally effective but without toxic side effects. And better still, after six months, only 10 percent of the exercise patients had relapsed, compared to 40 percent of the drug patients (Babyak et al. 2000). And most important, exercise can prevent cancer and its recurrence. An editorial in the *British Medical Journal* explored some of the reasons: exercise increases cardiovascular and lung capacity, balances hormone and energy levels, improves immune function, promotes bowel tone and motility, and supports DNA repair and antioxidant defense (Batty and Thune 2000).

Abundant research shows that physically active people have a lower incidence of cancer and cancer patients who exercise have a lower recurrence rate. Lance Armstrong is a famous example of how physical fitness and willpower can overcome the odds. A world-class athlete who won the Tour de France (a three-week 2,300 mile bicycle race through the mountains of France) seven times between 1999 and 2005, Armstrong was diagnosed in 1996 with testicular cancer that had metastasized to his lungs, abdomen, and brain. He used conventional treatment, fought the odds, and was later dubbed "the comeback kid." Armstrong has given the word "comeback" a whole new level of meaning in that he has not only survived cancer but also started competing professionally again in early 2009.

Research performed over twenty years ago showed that people who had been athletic in youth were less likely to get cancer later. The Harvard School of Public Health study showed that there was a lower incidence of breast and reproductive cancers in former college athletes. The breast-cancer risk was half that of nonathletes, and less than half for cancers of the reproductive organs (Frisch et al. 1985). One hypothesis related to this result is that physical activity uses hormones that could otherwise potentially drive cancerous growth, hormones that are necessary for growth and repair of normal tissues but aren't available for abnormal growth during exercise.

Even if you weren't an athlete in your youth, exercise is still beneficial. A study of over 4,000 women compared breast-cancer risk between a group of women who exercised and women in a sedentary control group (Holmes et al. 2005). Women with the highest levels of activity showed the greatest benefit. Exercise reduced breast-cancer risk by 20 to 40 percent, and the risk of larger and more advanced tumors was remarkably reduced. The difference in risk was the same regardless of whether the women were overweight or postmenopausal, or had a family history of cancer. Even women who increased their activity after age fifty had a 27 percent lower risk (Bardia et al. 2006).

## Cell Oxygenation

Nobel laureate Dr. Otto Warburg was mentioned in chapter 1 because he first identified the role of oxygen in cancer development. He discovered that a 35 percent decrease in cellular oxidation promotes cancer development (Warburg 1966). Exercise aerates the body at the cellular level as well as the circulation. This increased activity sweeps out the body at the deepest levels possible, relieving congestion caused by accumulated waste products, which devitalize the cells. For example, we feel sore when we exercise unused muscles because of lactic-acid drainage, and once it clears away, we're no longer sore. When the cellular environment is congested, nutrients are delivered to the cell less efficiently, and waste products accumulate. Lower oxygen availability to the cells can also be a factor in metastasis (Brizel et al. 1996), and exercise brings in more oxygen.

## Immunity

A study of AIDS patients clearly showed the effects of exercise on stress and immunity. Of course, AIDS patients' immune systems are already damaged or under attack from the HIV retrovirus. The study took place in HIV-positive patients who had just been diagnosed and were therefore at an extremely acute stage of stress. NK cell activity was measured in two groups, because it decreases with stress and trauma so reliably that it can be considered a marker for stress's effect on immunity. NK cell activity is also a marker for longevity in AIDS patients. The subjects were divided into two groups, one remaining inactive and the other exercising forty-five minutes three times a week. In the inactive group, NK cell activity declined, as anticipated. After one month, the group that exercised showed no decrease in NK cell activity, and other types of immune cells that normally drop increased. Exercise was a powerful coping mechanism for the stress of a devastating diagnosis but also a therapeutic countermeasure against the disease (LaPerriere et al. 1990).

Exercise also activates another type of immune cell, called the *macrophage*, which means "big eater." Macrophages engulf bacteria or various waste products and metabolic debris, and break them down. Activation of macrophages helps keep the internal environment sanitary and prevent infections from taking hold (Silveira et al. 2007). Macrophages help NK cells "clean up" the debris of destroyed cancer cells or microbes. Besides activating macrophages, exercise temporarily raises body temperature, which can kill germs and destroy cancer cells. It also reduces stress-related hormones like cortisol that lower activity of cells like NK cells and macrophages. You've already learned about the relationship between stress and the cancer-promoting factors of low immunity and inflammation; with less stress, there's less inflammation and more immune strength.

## Inflammation

As discussed, inflammation can be a driving force in cancer development. Exercise can directly decrease inflammation. Though the mechanism is likely complex, various research reports show that exercise can reduce C-reactive protein, IL-6, and NF-$k$B levels, all of which drive the inflammatory process (Kasapis and Thompson 2005).

# EXERCISE SUPPORTS A CANCER-PREVENTIVE PHYSIOLOGY

Exercise also appears to prevent abnormal angiogenesis. Although it hasn't been thoroughly researched, it's thought that by stimulating normal growth and repair, exercise inhibits the conditions that cause abnormal growth. A study published by BioMed Central in January 2004 reports that exercise increases production of the chemical that stops new blood vessel formation (angiogenesis) (Gu et al. 2004). Exercise also prevents oxidative stress, a major factor in aging and cancer development. Moderate exercise and endurance training, in which incremental increases in physical activity allow the body to strengthen gradually, don't stimulate inflammation or oxidative stress (Oztasan et al. 2004). A substantial anticancer benefit of exercise is that it stimulates the production of coenzyme $Q_{10}$, which, as previously mentioned, is an antioxidant that's used as a supplement and has shown substantial benefits in cancer treatment (Lockwood et al. 1994).

Exercise in cancer patients has been criticized because it's thought that cancer patients, who often suffer from fatigue, should rest and save their vital resources for healing. The most recent trend, however, supports having cancer patients exercise for therapeutic reasons, to improve the effects of treatment, and recovery time and treatment side effects, and to treat fatigue itself (Sood and Moynihan 2005).

# EXERCISE AND RECOVERY TIME FROM CANCER TREATMENT

Now that there's substantial scientific research to support exercise as a therapeutic and preventive cancer-fighting activity, knowledgeable experts no longer say to rest and conserve your strength. There are certainly times when rest is important, such as just after treatment, whether it's surgery, chemotherapy, or radiation. Recovery time between exercise activities is important too, especially if you were inactive in the past.

As mentioned, research shows that people who are generally very physically active are less prone to cancer in the first place. Not only does exercise increase survival time, even at late stages, but studies show a significantly lower rate of relapse for colon cancer (Meyerhardt et al. 2006). Likewise with prostate cancer, physically active men are less likely to get a cancer diagnosis and more likely to live longer if they do have cancer (Patel et al. 2005). Furthermore exercise seems to act at a deep level, affecting cellular chemistry (Leung et al. 2004).

Among female cancers, breast and ovarian cancers have been shown to respond well to exercise, with lower risk and longer survival time in both young and older women (Holmes et al. 2005; Cottreau, Ness, and Kriska 2000).

The benefits of exercise have also been studied in the context of lifestyle reform. You'll recall that we previously mentioned Dean Ornish's study of the combination of diet, exercise, and stress reduction (see the introduction). The blood of the men who had undergone lifestyle change was found to have a seven times greater inhibiting effect on cancer-cell growth in the laboratory (Ornish et al. 2005). Similar research has repeated these results and shown that one way that diet and exercise works is through its effect of reducing levels of insulin-like growth factor (Fontana, Klein, and Holloszy 2006), which we know promotes cancer. This same type of research was also performed with women, and tested on breast-cancer cells in a laboratory dish (Barnard et al. 2006).

# WHAT'S THE BEST KIND OF EXERCISE?

Exercise is defined very broadly. In some studies, exercise consisted of walking three times a week. In others, the exercise was aerobic, wherein the person exercising experiences a significantly increased heart rate and feels out of breath. Yet there's another category of exercise: mild, or "mindful," exercise, such as yoga and tai chi, both of which have roots in antiquity, but their benefits are measurable and have been studied for decades. Aerobic exercise can also be mindful, as anyone who has played tennis or handball can tell you, but merely in an external way. Aerobic exercise has psychological benefits and powerfully cleanses the cells. The milder exercises also seem to offer effects at the cellular level, as well as profound psychological benefits. Effective exercise need not be strenuous. Consistency is the most important factor. A brisk walk for thirty minutes five days a week reduces breast-cancer risk by 20 percent, even in postmenopausal women and women at high risk for the disease (McTiernan et al. 2003). Bicycle riding, swimming, hiking, or other moderate physical activity could be used as well.

## Mindful Exercise

**Yoga:** Though there are many types of yoga, hatha yoga, which involves stretching and holding various postures called *asanas*, is synonymous with yoga practice in the United States. Increasing your flexibility clears out the congestion and crystallized waste around the tendons and muscles. When this accumulated waste, mostly lactic acid, drains out, that familiar soreness we get when starting most types of exercise can be painful and stressful initially, but in hatha yoga, these side effects are greatly diminished. The stress-reducing effects of yoga are well known, and it even helps depression and offers many of the benefits of aerobic exercise (Woolery et al. 2004).

**Tai Chi:** A series of dance-like movements passed on from antiquity in China, tai chi chuan is also the basis for several martial arts forms. Tai chi has been extensively studied in China for its therapeutic properties and is often used for hospital patients with chronic disease (Sandlund and Norlander 2000).

**Qigong:** Though less pronounced in most of its forms, qigong, another Chinese gentle martial art, also requires movements. The main characteristic of the many styles of qigong is the cultivation of a qualitative sense of the body's vital energy. East Asian philosophy teaches that vital energy is a primary force of nature from which forms emerge, while Western science considers it to be the product of complex biochemical reactions. Regardless of where vital energy comes from, the art of qigong is to learn to feel it and build its force through movement, breath, and intention.

Like tai chi, qigong is used therapeutically in Chinese hospitals and is a fundamental part of cancer treatment in some locations. Many papers have reported the beneficial effects of qigong through stimulation of the immune system (Chen and Yeung 2002). Research has shown a measurable benefit in the increased production of interferon, a cytokine with antiviral and anticancer properties. In a study of 80 cancer patients, 25 were given chemotherapy only, 25 were given chemotherapy and qigong training, and 30 were given qigong training alone (ibid.). The group that practiced qigong as the sole treatment had increased red and white blood cells, and hemoglobin. The group given chemotherapy and qigong had increased red blood cells, blood platelets, and hemoglobin. White cells were not as high in the group whose sole treatment was qigong. The group that had chemotherapy only had a significant decrease in red and white blood cells, platelets, and hemoglobin.

## Don't Like to Exercise? Try to Have Fun

If exercise doesn't sound like fun to you, join a group. Social activities encourage regular activity. If you have a tennis partner or volleyball team, you're obligated to show up, which is easier than the "tough love" approach of self-discipline. Even having a jogging partner can relieve the monotony of regular activity. If you hate exercise, it's essential to have group support and plan "exercise dates" to keep you moving.

## How Much Exercise Do You Need?

Regularly performed moderate physical activity presents a number of benefits to your whole organism, especially regarding immune-system functioning, such as augmenting resistance to infections and cancer growth. Too much effort or strain has the obvious risk of injury, but it can also disrupt the cellular antioxidant system. Another reason to go slowly at first is that you might provoke a "detox" reaction. If built-up waste in the connective tissues is suddenly mobilized, the resulting malaise can resemble a case of the flu, which will pass, of course, but it may delay your effort to start regular exercise while you recover.

Do you suffer from fatigue? If you're fatigued from cancer, chemotherapy, or both, it may seem nonsensical to suggest exercise rather than more rest, but cancer experts now claim that exercise is the most reliable treatment for fatigue. Starting with two to three minutes, even very weak cancer patients can often increase to twenty-five to thirty minutes of moderate exercise (such as using a treadmill) within two to three months.

It's important to figure out how much activity is right for you. If you want to enjoy the advantages of aerobic exercise, you don't have to commit a lot of time. Most people can spare at least ten minutes a day. In only ten minutes, your body and metabolism can function at a higher level, with effects that last for twenty-four hours at first, and improved benefits with daily activity (Hansen, Stevens, and Coast 2001).

To find your optimum heart rate for beginning exercise, measure your resting heart rate by checking your pulse at your wrist or neck and counting the beats in one minute. Subtract this number from 220 and then multiply this number by half. Then add the number of beats in the resting heart rate again. This number is the number of beats per minute at the low end of your target heart rate. For example, if your resting heart rate is 70 beats per minute, then 220 minus 80 equals 140. Half of 140 is 70. Add the resting heart rate of 70 to 70, and the target heart rate is 140 beats per minute. To find the high end, use three quarters in place of one half. In this case we calculate that 220 minus 80 equals 140. Three fourths of 140 is 105. You add the resting heart rate value of 80 to 105 to get the high-end target heart rate of 185. You can measure your heart rate by checking your pulse at your wrist or neck, but it's easier to use a heart monitor if you want to check it every day. Some sporting goods and electronics stores offer small portable ones. This method of monitoring your exercise is good for general purposes, health maintenance, and stress reduction. If you have any medical concerns, be sure to work out your exercise program with your doctor or a professional referred by your doctor. If you're exercising for prevention, you can approach it with fewer constrictions.

Another way to measure your degree of physical activity is the *metabolic equivalent task* (*MET*). Many recommendations for physical activity are classified as "light," "medium," or "vigorous," with subclassifications in between. Vigorous exercise for one person may be light for another. It depends on how hard you have to work at it, which varies from one person to another. One MET hour is the energy (oxygen) used by the body when sitting quietly. The more vigorous the activity, the greater the number of MET hours, and the number of MET hours is the measure of intensity of physical activity (Ainsworth et al. 2000).

# PHYSICAL ACTIVITY IN METS (METABOLIC EQUIVALENT TASKS)

| Activity | MET Hours | Activity | MET Hours |
|---|---|---|---|
| **Very Light** | | Vigorous | |
| Walking (taking a stroll) | 2 | Skating | 6 |
| | | Doubles tennis, more running | 7 |
| Playing a musical instrument | 2 | Hiking | 6–7 |
| **Light** | | Swimming laps | 6–8 |
| Walking at a normal pace | 2½–3 | Rowing, canoeing, kayaking vigorously | 6–8 |
| Slow dancing | 2½–3 | Dancing (vigorous) | 6–8 |
| Golfing (using an electric golf cart) | 2½–3 | Some exercise apparatuses | 6–8 |
| Bowling | 2½–3 | Bicycling (10 to 16 mph) | 6–10 |
| **Slightly Vigorous** | | | |
| Brisk walking (3 mph) | 3½ | Swimming laps moderately fast | 6–10 |
| Weight lifting | 3½ | Aerobic calisthenics | 6–10 |
| Water aerobics | 3½ | Squash, racquetball, handball, tennis | 7–12 |
| Canoeing, kayaking | 3½ | | |
| Climbing stairs | 4 | Jogging (1 mile every 12 min.) | 8 |
| Dancing | 4 | | |
| Bicycling | 4 | Skiing (downhill or cross-country) | 8 |
| **Moderately Vigorous** | | Running 6 mph (10-min. mile) | 10 |
| Swimming | 4½ | | |
| Golf, carrying clubs | 4½ | Running 8 mph (7.5-min. mile) | 14 |
| Doubles tennis | 5 | | |
| Exercise machines | 5 | Running 10 mph (6-min. mile) | 16 |
| Slow jogging | 5 | | |
| Fast dancing | 5 | | |

Based on data from "Compendium of Physical Activities: An Update of Activity Codes and MET Intensities," by B. E. Ainsworth, W. L. Haskell, M. C. Whitt, M. L. Irwin, A. M. Swartz, S. J. Strath, W. L. O'Brien, D. R. Bassett Jr., K. H. Schmitz, P. O. Emplaincourt, D. R. Jacobs Jr., and A. S. Leon, in *Medicine and Science in Sports and Exercise* 32 (Suppl. 9):S498–516, 2000.

To calculate your weekly MET hours, multiply each activity you participated in by the number of hours spent each time, and then add all of them. For example:

Dancing (vigorously) 2 hours: 7 x 2 = 14 METs

Walking (rapidly) 4 hours: 3.5 x 4 = 14 METs

Playing tennis 1 hour: 8 METs

Total: 36 METs for the week

As a general rule, when the cancer is deeper in the body, more exercise is necessary to activate the tissue layers. It takes longer for the blood circulation to activate deep in the abdomen, compared to in the muscles, skin, or areas near the skin's surface. Optimal activity for breast cancer requires at least 9 METs a week (Holmes et al. 2005). Colon cancer requires twice as much at 18 METs a week (Pratap and Schroy III 2007). Prostate cancer buried deep in the groin requires more activity at 30 METs a week (Giovannucci et al. 1998a). The minimum recommendation for a protective effect favors moderate activity at a minimum of 4.5 METs. Less than 4.5 METs has a significantly reduced effect (Thune and Furberg 2001).

## Exercises to Avoid

Always speak with your doctor before starting an exercise program, and make sure that you avoid exercises or activities not recommended by your doctor. Bouncing on a trampoline-type rebounder is not recommended if you have lymphoma or lymphocytic leukemia. Though an excellent tool for aerobic exercise, rebounders are used to stimulate lymph circulation, so you should discuss their use with your physician as a precaution (Bhattacharya et al. 1980). Avoid vigorous arm movements after surgical removal of lymph nodes from the armpits, and don't jog if you have bone metastases. You may have to limit your activity if you

*Success with an Integrative Strategy*

P. A., aged sixty, was diagnosed with a malignant tumor in her left breast with several malignant nodes. After lumpectomy and node removal, she worked with her acupuncturist to develop a comprehensive diet and lifestyle program. Though her doctors didn't push for chemotherapy, they strongly recommended radiation treatment. She refused radiation but followed up with mammograms every six months. Because she and her husband were close friends with several doctors, she was still monitored as she embarked on her treatment plan. The anxiety from the cancer diagnosis was severe, with a high level of fear of recurrence. Her main weapon against the anxiety was a vigorous exercise program, including gym workouts and lots of bicycling. She spent at least two hours a day on at least two forms of exercise. The vigorous exercise gave her the emotional steadiness to include yoga in the evenings, and she emphasized yoga and meditation during the winter, when running and cycling were less practical. Along with her diet program and strategic use of supplements, her sense of well-being and confidence improved to the extent that her emotional agitation and fear of recurrence disappeared.

have anemia, low white-cell count, or low platelet levels. Symptoms such as dizziness or loss of balance, chest pain, heart arrhythmia, tachycardia, leg cramps, or wheezing may restrict the type and amount of exercise you can do. Current National Center on Physical Activity and Disability cancer guidelines (2009) recommend avoiding exercise within two hours of chemotherapy or radiation therapy, since increases in circulation may increase the effects of the treatments. You might want to learn to monitor your heart rate, rhythm, and blood pressure after exercise, especially if your body gets "revved up" and feels as if it's straining after a short period of exercise or if you're struggling with fatigue.

## ASSESS THE AMOUNT OF EXERCISE YOU GET

Circle "Y" for yes or "N" for no, and mark in the number of points indicated for each question:

Y or N   _____   Are you overweight (if yes, subtract 1 point)?

Y or N   _____   Do you work out at a gym (if yes, add 1 point)?

Y or N   _____   Do you play a sport regularly (if yes, add 1 point)?

Y or N   _____   How many hours a week do you exercise (if 6 hours, add 1 point; if 12 hours, add 2 points; and if 16 hours or more, add 3 points)?

A total of two points or fewer means that you would benefit from more physical activity.

# CHAPTER 9

# Emotional Healing

Don't underrate the importance of emotional healing. Gritting your teeth and suffering silently may have a price: the sacrifice of your immunity and your enjoyment of life. Dealing with your emotions can be the most difficult part of the journey. While it may not be easy to change your diet or start exercising, facing up to your buried traumas and negative experiences, and their residual effects can be the biggest challenge of all. Nevertheless emotional healing can not only lengthen your life but also make you really glad to be alive.

Emotional healing means to bring a sense of well-being into our lives for the purpose of improving our emotional and physical health. Recent research shows that happiness reduces inflammation. According to a 2008 study in England (Steptoe et al. 2008), a positive mood reduces the level of the stress hormone cortisol, which is associated not only with increased risk of heart disease and cancer but also many other types of disease: allergies, asthma, arthritis, and cardiovascular disease, to name a few common examples. The study also found that positive moods are associated with other inflammatory markers, such as C-reactive protein and the pro-inflammatory cytokine IL-6.

Stressful events are the main triggers for the negative emotions that cause emotional distress, but the most important factor for long-term health is to realize that we actually "store up" negative emotions and past traumas. If we don't resolve these stored traumas, they can cause negative attitudes and expectations that become self-fulfilling. Old patterns recorded in the brain and nervous system can make us react according to old conflicts and painful memories, recreating old dramas again and again in new situations and reinforcing a false, negative view of ourselves (Bremner et al. 1993).

This chapter discusses the importance of trauma and how it has been an underrated factor as a cause of disease, and explains its effects on the immune system and on chronic inflammation. It also explains how to heal the effects of trauma and offers several proven strategies. We will also discuss techniques for healing trauma; research on the use of journal writing, the methodology and health benefits of forgiveness, and the dangers of social isolation and guilt; and discussion about how addressing these areas helps achieve longevity and enhanced quality of life.

# TRAUMA

Trauma is a severely stressful event, or even repeated stressful events, from which you haven't had time to recover. We're all trauma victims; as human beings, we all suffer, as Shakespeare's Hamlet expressed it, "the thousand natural shocks that flesh is heir to." There's no black-and-white boundary between people who are hurting from a past traumatic experience and those who aren't. It's just a matter of degree. You may not have suffered a trauma as severe as physical assault or public humiliation, but we all have minor versions of trauma; the fight with a spouse, office politics, financial setbacks, and even surly store clerks can cause a small-scale trauma that requires hours or days, but not years, to recover from. If you or a loved one has had a cancer diagnosis, you know about trauma. Severe traumas can take years to recover from, even with treatment. The symptoms of minor traumas are similar to those of severe ones, but they clear up more rapidly. Let's look at specific characteristics some people have after exposure to a severe traumatic stressor, usually from direct personal experience of an event involving actual or threatened death or serious injury, or some other threat to one's physical person, including diagnosis of a life-threatening illness; this condition is known as *post-traumatic stress disorder (PTSD)*.

## PTSD

What can we learn about stress and trauma from those who suffer from it in its most extreme form? PTSD is characterized by symptoms such as guilt about surviving a life-threatening event when others didn't, guilt about having somehow caused the traumatic event, reliving the traumatic event in dreams, apathy, emotional numbness, a sense of dreamlike detachment from involvement with reality, hypervigilance, panic attacks, and recurrent trauma-related thoughts and images. Those with a severe case of PTSD can't seem to put their lives back together, and need professional help, as well as the support of friends and family.

# CHARACTERISTICS OF PTSD

| Psychological: | Emotional: | Behavioral: | Physical: |
| --- | --- | --- | --- |
| Lack of concentration | Depression and loss of meaning | Hyperarousal, irritability, agitation | Chest tightness, palpitations |
| Poor judgment, indecision | Withdrawal (hiding feelings) | Insomnia, shallow sleep with nightmares | Stomach and digestive problems |
| Hypervigilance (agitated state of arousal) | Intense fear, panic | Withdrawal (physical isolation) | Spontaneous perspiration |
| Intrusive thoughts and memories | Feelings of helplessness, self-criticism | Substance abuse | Hyperventilation |
| | | | Immunosuppression |

## LONG-TERM EFFECTS OF PTSD

Reduced NK cell activity appears to correlate strongly with the lingering mental and physical effects of PTSD. PTSD can have a *long-term* impact on health since it's known to suppress immunity even for years. NK (natural killer) cell activity may be a key factor in chronic disease as well as an important link in mind-body medicine. Loss of immunity in the form of inhibition of the *scavenging* function of NK cells and macrophages may be a significant factor in the origin of such diseases as cancer, hepatitis, diabetes, chronic infections, opportunistic infections, and even autoimmune diseases (Hogan and Basten 1988).

# Trauma and Immunity

Stress and trauma's adverse effect on the immune system is now well established. The leading cause of "late death" after a traumatic event is *infection* (Ader, Felton, and Cohen 2000); this means that if the person didn't die from the original trauma, often within weeks of the traumatic event, the person will die from a disease like pneumonia from a weakened immune system. Numerous immune and nervous system, and hormonal changes occur in response to stressful events or circumstances, but one common reaction in the immune system is reduced NK cell activity. This is an important mind-body link in medical science. NK cell function is influenced by a wide variety of stressors, including physical injury caused by accidents, surgery, and other medical treatments (Koga et al. 2001); nutritional deficiencies; emotional trauma;

### Trauma, Stress, and NK Cell Activity

NK cell activity is reduced by:

> Physical trauma, including surgery and various medical interventions

> Nutritional deficiencies

> Stress from natural disasters

> Depression, anxiety, and fatigue

> Nervous system and adrenal arousal, flight-or-fight conditions

grief; and hormone imbalances. Victims of disasters such as hurricanes and earthquakes show lower NK cell activity (Ironson et al. 1997; Inoue-Sakurai, Maruyama, and Morimoto 2000).

Negative psychological states such as depression, anxiety, and fatigue can also affect NK cell activity, even if lymphocyte counts don't change. Negative psychological states such as self-consciousness and self-criticism have also been shown to decrease NK cell activity (Christensen et al. 1996).

NK cell activity is also used as an index of survival time. Doctors at the National Cancer Institute (NCI) have measured NK cell activity test results to determine the survival prognosis in AIDS and cancer patients (Levy et al. 1985). Feelings of helplessness may also lower NK cell activity. Similar to how the laboratory test rats, mentioned earlier, that couldn't escape from random stressful stimuli suffered the most, researchers studying breast-cancer patients found that those who felt depressed and helpless had lower NK cell activity than those with the psychological resilience to cope with the disease (Levy et al. 1987).

## EARLY TRAUMA

Evidence suggests that early adverse experiences play a preeminent role in development of mood and anxiety disorders and that a brain hormone is the mediator. A persistent sensitizing of the nervous system and adrenal glands, even to mild stress in adulthood, causes predisposition to mental and emotional health problems (Heim et al. 2000). Old psychological wounds set up an exaggerated stress response that can contribute to the growth and spread of cancer (Reiche, Nunes, and Morimoto 2004).

## Trauma, Stress, and Inflammation

As you've learned, stress and trauma have well-established effects on immunity. It's also now established that stress causes hormonal and immune system changes that activate or exaggerate the body's inflammatory response. Accumulated stress can increase production of pro-inflammatory chemicals like IL-6 (Costanzo et al. 2005), which we know promotes the growth and development of tumors, so stress is a significant factor in the origination and development of cancer (Black 2003). Early trauma can be a factor in chronically impaired immunity. In sensitized early trauma patients, the inflammatory reaction to stress can be particularly intense, and the culprit here is NF-*k*B, the pro-inflammatory factor that contributes to cancer development (Pace et al. 2006).

Stress can also induce changes in the blood vessel formation process (Thaker et al. 2006), and you've learned how factors that promote angiogenesis also promote cancer. Chronic stress is probably a causal factor for many diseases as well as for a shorter survival time.

## Cancer, Trauma, and Depression

As discussed, in recent years the relationship between the effects of stress and trauma have been correlated with numerous types of health problems, including cancer development. You've also learned how trauma, especially early in life, can be related to chronic health problems. Research into personality types points toward a certain temperament that may be more prone to cancer than others. People who are the cancer type, or "type C," don't complain, and suffer willingly. They don't easily express anger, they try to conform to others' expectations, and they often suffer feelings of helplessness in the face of stressful triggers (Temoshok 1987). Many people diagnosed with cancer believe that it was caused by a traumatic event, which naturally results in feelings of guilt or that this life-threatening condition was brought on by circumstances that could or should have been under their control: a divorce, job loss, alienation of one's children, or any number of personal catastrophes. This guilt or feeling of failure, whether rational or not, can be the worst symptom.

Depression is correlated with shortened survival time in cancer. In mind-body medicine, depression correlates with inflammation, driven by inflammatory cytokines like IL-6, which could be one of the reasons why chronic stress seems to promote tumor growth, but the inflammatory cytokines themselves may induce feelings of despair and hopelessness and play a role in cancer-related fatigue (Tchekmedyian et al. 2003) in a kind of feedback loop that can spiral downward into despair and accelerated deterioration in physical symptoms (Illman et al. 2005).

Despite these findings, there's still no clear-cut evidence that trauma, stress, or a certain personality type is actually a direct *cause* of cancer, though it may be a contributing factor. A severe stressful event can be thought of as a trigger rather than a cause. The only *proven* causes of cancer are toxic influences, such as certain chemical poisons and radiation. Even though a stressful event causes changes in the body's physiology that can promote cancer development, internal conditions must be "ripe" to develop into cancer. It's necessary to maintain a good internal condition through our lifestyle habits so that we're less vulnerable to the inevitable shocks and stresses that life brings.

Trauma and chronic stress can lower immunity and help cultivate an internal condition that can develop into cancer by promoting inflammation and angiogenesis. Diet and supplementation may not be sufficient to boost immunity if the stress burden is too cumbersome.

# HEALING PATHS FOR DEALING WITH EMOTIONS

Given the strong connection among cancer, trauma, and chronic stress, what can you do to fight cancer effectively and prevent its recurrence? Here are the key elements of a treatment plan:

> **Get support.** Work with a physician you can talk to who supports your desire to avoid any unnecessary medical intervention. Get support from family; friends; or members of any religious, service, or social organizations you belong to.

> **Strengthen your immunity.** Become a pleasure seeker in the sense of building relaxation and entertainment into your life.

> **Get nurturing treatment.** Consult a massage therapist for professional nurturing bodywork, or have someone you know give you a shoulder rub, allowing yourself to do nothing except passively receive relaxing touch for stress relief.

> **Get desensitizing treatment.** Consult a practitioner of one of several specialized treatments to help you access and process buried emotional patterns and traumas, and diminish their impact on you.

> **Express yourself.** Take classes or undergo therapies in which you're guided though a process of self-expression.

## Get Support

Because the healing process is multifaceted, it's hard to do it alone. Cultivating a support network is an important part of the process that should be considered with care and planning. Professional help; personal, emotional, and intellectual support; and the ability to talk to people who've traveled this road before are all necessary.

**Medical Support for Emotional Heath:** It's not only important to confront the reality of negative emotions, including anxiety and depression, but also to keep your spirits up and avoid descending too deeply into your suffering. Use drugs for depression and mood disorders with caution, because they're only a partial solution, at best, and require careful monitoring by your prescribing professional. Discuss this issue with your physician, getting a second opinion, if possible, as well as with your family. Work with a doctor who's willing to help you get off the drugs as soon as possible and who will prescribe drugs that are easy to stop taking without severe side effects.

Antidepressant drugs aren't as effective as commonly thought, according to a review by U.S. and Canadian researchers (Kirsch et al. 2008), who reported that patients taking the drugs didn't improve any more than those taking a placebo. The exception to this was the severely depressed patients, who improved more on the drugs than the placebos, but only slightly. This report, created for submission to the FDA, used a vaster data set than a typical study does. The researchers found that the overall effect of antidepressant medication isn't as clinically significant as previously thought, reporting that the new generation of antidepressants doesn't produce clinically significant improvements in depression in patients who initially have moderate or even very severe depression compared to a placebo, but show significant effects only in the most severely depressed patients. The important point is to use drugs only for crisis management or as a last resort, such as in cases of severe symptoms.

A survey published in *Consumer Reports* (Metcalf 2004) revealed that the side effects of antidepressants (including suicidal longings) are more common than previously stated in the package inserts, and reported: "A combination of talk therapy and drugs worked best for treatment of depression and anxiety. But those whose treatment consisted of mostly talk therapy did almost as well if they had thirteen or more visits with the therapist." Talk therapy is underrated, because drugs are more prominent in the public's awareness. But talk therapy takes time and isn't an instant cure. Real healing seldom involves an instant cure. If you see a psychiatrist, you're more likely to get medication, but psychologists, social workers, and counselors can often provide effective talk therapy.

Likewise, drugs for treatment of PTSD, especially *selective serotonin reuptake inhibitors* (*SSRIs*), are said to reduce symptoms by half or less, but many of the common beliefs about these drugs are in question. Some studies have shown that they're no more effective than a placebo (Antonuccio et al. 1999). They also can cause unsettling side effects, such as loss of libido (Labbate 1999). There's also encouraging evidence that if drugs are used within days after a trauma, they can prevent the occurrence of PTSD symptoms (Zohar et al. 2009). For long-term treatment, evidence shows that psychotherapy is more effective than drugs (Berger et al. 2009). It's worth the time and effort to seek professional talk therapy to confront fear, sadness, and anything else that deprives you of your sense of worth or well-being, or enjoyment of life (Solomon, Gerrity, and Muff 1992). Several types of therapy interventions, including both individual counseling and group therapy, seem to help reduce psychological suffering.

**Supportive Relationships:** One research study (Price et al. 2001) shows that the risk of developing breast cancer is as much as nine times higher in women with a combination of high stress and social isolation. So it's a good idea to create a caring network consisting not only of health care professionals but also social connections.

> **Family Support:** You can get emotional support from friends or coworkers, but they're rarely as helpful or consistent in meeting our needs as family. Nevertheless, every case differs; some people have an easier time talking to their friends than their family members.

> **Social Support:** Social support from friends can be a tremendously valuable comfort and resource. Getting support from friends is problematic for some

people with a cancer diagnosis, because "breaking the news" can be difficult. You want to continue to live "among the living" and avoid being stigmatized by a medical diagnosis and all of its assumed implications. You don't want to make friends feel uncomfortable around you and have your diagnosis become your new identity. Though a difficult burden, it's your responsibility to put your friends at ease by talking about your condition easily and comfortably. Here's where a sense of humor helps, but successful communication depends on openness and clarity in asking for what you want from your friends, such as permission to freely discuss your feelings with them, and agreement about whom to tell the news and who you'd prefer not know.

> **Pet Therapy:** Pets can be a great source of comfort and can increase your sense of purpose and devotion to life in all its forms; evidence suggests that keeping pets can increase life span (Brickel 1980).

## Strengthen Your Immunity

While there are various ways to stimulate NK cell activity, learning what makes you happy is the major part of the solution. In a Japanese study, music therapy was observed to increased NK cell activity and count (Hasegawa et al. 2001), and daily massage increased NK cell activity and count in another study (Ironson et al. 1986).

Lifestyle, as well as stress, affects NK cell activity. Research correlates a healthy lifestyle with significantly higher NK cell and other immune cell activity (Kusaka, Kondou, and Morimoto 1992). The lifestyle factors evaluated assessed study participants on hours of sleep, exercise time, hours of work, mental stress, type of diet, breakfast habits, and alcohol or tobacco consumption. Using certain antioxidants, such as the amino acids NAC (n-acetylcysteine) and thioproline, vitamin E, and, to some extent, vitamin C, as well as AHCC, also appear to activate NK cells (Ferrández et al. 1999). Toxic lifestyle habits, on the other hand, can reduce NK cell activity and immune resistance (Nair, Kronfol, and Schwartz 1990). Remember that coffee (Ulvik et al. 2008) and sugar (Wyshak and Frisch 1994) can deplete vital resources like B vitamins and calcium.

## Get Nurturing Treatments

Regular stress reduction trains the body to react to stress with less intensity and gets the pleasure (and pain-relieving) neurotransmitters (endorphins) flowing. The effect may be only temporary at first, but continuing to get stress-reducing treatments will acquaint you with a "new" but familiar you. A lot of treatment methods are available, so the best starting point is from within your own personal network, perhaps through a friend's or health care provider's recommendation. Next it's important to evaluate the rapport between you and the practitioner.

A practitioner may have an excellent reputation, but if you don't feel that you have a good relationship with that person, then it's not a good match.

**Massage and Structural Therapy:** Also called *bodywork*, massage therapy focuses on relaxing and releasing the accumulated tension in the muscles and tendons. Sophisticated methods to restructure your body and restore the relationship between the nerves and muscles are also available. A lot of these methods can help with old injuries and chronic problems by retraining the body's customary and often uncomfortable patterns. Some of the better-known techniques include the Rolf Method of Structural Integration (also known as Rolfing), which once had a reputation as a painful, deep massage; however, most people today find it very relaxing and non-intrusive (www.rolf.org). The Feldenkrais Method, named after its founder, Moshe Feldenkrais, whose diverse background included work as a physicist, engineer, and martial artist, reorganizes how the nerves stimulate the muscles. During a session, the technique may seem very subtle, but the results after one session are often striking (www.feldenkrais.com). Craniosacral therapy is a variety of techniques that center on gentle, nonforceful adjustments of the cranium and the spine. The various techniques work on both the nervous system and the muscular tissues, based on osteopathic methods (www.bodyenergy.net). Massage therapy not only relieves the stress cancer patients suffer but also strengthens the immune response. Massage can improve the immune system's ability to destroy cancer cells (Ironson et al. 1986; Hernandez-Reif et al. 2005). Check with your doctor about the advisability of massage if you're undergoing cancer treatment.

People often find that releasing muscular tension can also release stored emotional tension, which can be a valuable complement to other types of therapy. Some schools of psychotherapy are even based on this principle. Some massage therapists are also oriented to assisting their clients with emotional release. The key is to work with someone you trust and, if it all seems overwhelming, get more help if you need it.

**Acupuncture:** Best known for pain relief (Patel et al. 1989), acupuncture is also excellent for any stress-related condition. One mechanism proposed for the pain-relieving effect is that the needle stimulation causes the brain to release the body's natural opiates, endorphins (Clement-Jones et al. 1980). As previously mentioned, these brain chemicals induce a sense of well-being and are associated with "runner's high," though they're stimulated by many types of influences and suppressed by stress.

Does it hurt? The needle stimulation itself is usually very slight. The needles are often as fine as hairs and have a tapered point, which doesn't create such a sharp sensation. The acupuncture needle isn't hollow and doesn't cut the skin, unlike the much larger injection needle used in medical clinics.

**Biofeedback:** Biofeedback trains the brain to slow brain waves down to a calm, or *alpha*, state, and also monitors other stress responses so that the person undergoing treatment is trained to calm down to a lower level of reactivity. With sufficient practice, a person can also learn to invoke the alpha state at will.

## Get Desensitizing Treatment

After an overpowering stressful event, such as physical trauma, death of a loved one, or some other loss, it's normal to suppress some or most of your feelings around the incident, or even to "go numb." When major stress or any part of it is suppressed, it still exists as unconscious anguish and continues to affect how we feel and function day to day, manipulating our actions from "behind the scenes." The suppressed feelings become, in effect, a buried negative program. To *deprogram* these emotions, we must locate them and bring them to consciousness. Otherwise they can become the cause of nightmares or obsessive, intrusive memories. Painful memories can never be forgotten, but you can desensitize to them so that they no longer have control over your life. If you have painful memories or trauma, even early childhood trauma, it's possible to process it and regain a sense of control over your life and destiny. People with cancer, and even those who've recovered from cancer, sometimes have an obsessive fixation on their diagnosis that can be unhealthy and disempowering. Sometimes, regaining your power requires an outside intervention; sometimes you need a professional to help you access buried emotions. If you could access them yourself, they wouldn't be buried. If these emotions were conscious, they wouldn't be *unconscious*. Several techniques are available to help resolve this type of problem.

**Eye Movement Desensitization and Reprocessing (EMDR):** While EMDR (www.emdr.com) sounds strange when you first hear of it, the practitioner directs your eye movements while leading you in a structured therapy protocol. In this method *desensitization* refers to relieving a trauma's impact on the nervous system (Davidson and Parker 2001). The emotional wound may remain, but if desensitization is successful, it's no longer "raw." In 2004 the Department of Veterans Affairs and Department of Defense rated EMDR in their "A" category, meaning that it's strongly recommended for use in PTSD treatment (Veterans Health Administration and Department of Defense 2004). One Iraq War veteran, who'd been attacked by enemy fire and seen his buddies killed, suffered severe PTSD that included panic attacks, frequent horrific nightmares, and hallucinations of the smell of smoke and sight of blood. After several sessions of EMDR, he told me, "I'll never forget what I saw and felt, but it has lost its grip on me; it doesn't run my life anymore."

**Emotional Freedom Technique (EFT):** Like EMDR, Emotional Freedom Technique (EFT) (www.emofree.com) appear to have a reprogramming effect on the nervous system by giving it a physical cue. In this case, the cue is to tap on various points on the body. The practitioner helps you develop a type of "script" for your specific issues and needs, which the practitioner then recites while tapping on various points on your body, usually on the face, chest, and wrists. EFT's advantage is that you can practice it at home every day or several times a day once you've learned the protocol. You can then check in with the practitioner to see if your situation has changed such that your script needs revision. EFT have been helpful with substance abuse problems as severe as methamphetamine addiction and alcoholism.

**Somatic Experiencing (SE):** Biophysicist and psychologist Peter Levine developed Somatic Experiencing (www.traumahealing.com) specifically for trauma recovery. SE uses an awareness technique based on body sensations to help trauma victims "renegotiate" the traumas and their effects without attempting to recall or reexperience them. The technique provides an outlet for the pent-up "survival energies" to be expressed and discharged. As this occurs, people experience symptom relief and are able to return to normal life. The procedure, which isn't a type of hypnosis, is done in person in a session similar to psychotherapy. You delve into your experience as remembered by your senses. SE practitioners complete a thorough three-year training program before working with clients. In fewer than ten sessions, victims of severe sudden trauma ("shock trauma") experience relief from debilitating emotional and even physical symptoms. SE is also considered effective for early trauma, which usually requires longer-term treatment in conjunction with standard psychotherapy (Levine 1997).

**Holotropic Breathwork:** Holotropic Breathwork (http://holotropicbreathwork.ning.com and www.holotropic.com) is another technique in which a specially trained practitioner guides you through an emotional-release process. You're asked to follow the practitioner's guidance through a series of timed inhalations and exhalations. The practitioner guides you through the process by observing your responses, which provides access to your unconscious processes in a unique way. People often experience traumatic memories and feel them resolve with each breath. Most people find the process pleasant. You may later relive the trauma but in a new relationship to the symptoms and suffering.

## Express Yourself

Self-expression is especially important for the type C personality (serious, conscientious, orderly, and thrives on details and facts), but even if you aren't a classic type C, you may still have important things to express that, if left unexpressed, could hold you back from your ideal comfort level (Quartana, Laubmeier, and Zakowski 2006). It might be useful to have several means of self-expression; for example, one-on-one psychotherapy may be beneficial, especially if you lack family support. Support groups can also be valuable, because even with family support, it can be hard for family and friends to understand what it feels like to be in your situation, especially if you've received a cancer diagnosis. When you're with people who have to walk the same road, you can form powerful bonds, and insights from other people's experiences can have a profound, resonant effect.

**Psychotherapy:** During the healing process, it often helps to talk, sometimes to a professional, especially one who specializes in your issues (whether they include cancer diagnosis or war trauma) and who's willing to get to know you and understand your needs.

## Expressing Yourself Through Writing

Writing is an especially powerful tool for self-discovery, for achieving personal goals, and for cultivating peace of mind. It's a delusion to think that you can understand something clearly and still have a problem expressing it. The very process of writing down your thoughts requires clarifying them. Writing has its surprises too; for example, you may think you understand what's in your heart, but when you write from the heart, when you really try to write your feelings honestly and clearly, you may be amazed to read what comes out on the paper. Writing is a form of expression that involves both sides of the brain: the surprises may come from the intuitive right side, but they're filtered through language, which requires the linear left brain.

In a study reported in the *Oncologist* in February 2008 (Morgan et al. 2008), expressive writing, which involves writing down your deepest thoughts and feelings, may improve quality of life in cancer patients. Laboratory experiments with controls have already suggested that expressive writing helps physical and psychological well-being (Frisina, Borod, and Lepore 2004). This recent study (Morgan et al. 2008), conducted in the waiting rooms of an oncology clinic, confirmed the previous theoretical studies. The researchers found that journal writing positively affects the way patients think and feel about their illness. The researchers also analyzed the content of the patients' writings. Many patients wrote that the changes brought about in their lives by the cancer diagnosis were positive ones: that cancer had altered their views about family, spirituality, work, and the future. One patient wrote: "Don't get me wrong: cancer isn't a gift; it just showed me what the gifts in my life are."

**Support Group Therapy:** One of the keys to happiness is having authentic relationships. Early studies showed that support group therapy can lengthen survival time in cancer patients who were diagnosed as terminal, while other studies show no change in survival time but have established quality-of-life benefits (Kogon et al. 1997). So a well-run program with experienced group leaders could make a big difference (Clark, Bostwick, and Rummans 2003).

**Creative Expression:** Expressing yourself creatively is a matter of personal inclination. Writing, painting, acting, taking up photography, and any other means of artistic expression can yield psychological benefits beyond expectation. Creative movement, like ballroom dancing or modern dance, can support both physical fitness and creative expression.

The best therapy is to find your own way, to find your passion. Just because no one has researched the health benefits of ballroom dancing doesn't mean that they're not as powerful for you as anything else. Any creative and emotional outlet gives back what you put into it many times over.

Check around to see what's available in your area; there may be an array of interesting opportunities. I've known people who benefited from a variety of powerful activities that were provided on a small and local scale. I know people who've experienced healing from "painting from the unconscious" in a dimly lit classroom, wilderness survival training, model mugging (a self-defense class, usually requiring only a one-day or weekend training), trapeze training, skydiving, and karate training. You can fill your list with as many interests, hobbies, and fantasies as you can imagine.

## CHECKLIST: SIGNS OF EMOTIONAL STRESS:

| Emotional and Psychological Signs: | Physical Signs: |
|---|---|
| Sadness throughout the day, almost every day | Not enough sleep, sleep disturbances, or restless sleep |
| Loss of interest in or enjoyment of your favorite activities | Too much sugar |
| Loss of libido | Craving for drugs or alcohol |
| Feelings of emptiness or hopelessness | Constipation |
| Feeling nervous or overwhelmed | Pain |
| Trouble concentrating and making decisions | Fatigue or lack of energy |
| Feelings of worthlessness | Changes in appetite |
| Feelings of guilt | Body aches and pains |
| Irritability, restlessness | Sensitivity to stress and physical pain |
| Thoughts of death or suicide | |
| Intrusive thoughts and memories, nightmares | |

### ACCUMULATED STRESS

Circle "Y" for yes or "N" for no, and mark in one point for each yes answer:

Y or N    _____     Are you frequently in a bad mood?

Y or N    _____     Do you crave food, alcohol, or sweets every day?

Y or N    _____     Do you sleep poorly at night and still feel tired when you get up?

Y or N    _____     Are you easily irritated?

Y or N    _____     Have you ever had stomach or duodenal ulcers?

Y or N    _____     Have you ever had colitis or diverticulitis?

Y or N   _____    Have you had any automobile accidents within the last year (two points for this one)?

Y or N   _____    Have you had any other accidents, including sports injuries, within the last year?

## TRAUMAS

Circle "Y" for yes or "N" for no, and mark in three points for each yes answer:

Y or N   _____    Have you had a cancer diagnosis?

Y or N   _____    Have you lost a loved one within the last two years?

Y or N   _____    Do you have a loved one who's enduring a major illness?

Y or N   _____    Have you divorced or separated from your partner within the last two years?

Y or N   _____    Have you lost a job recently?

Y or N   _____    Have you had any surgery (other than dental) within the last year?

Y or N   _____    Have you been in military combat (five points for this one)?

A score of three points for accumulated stress or for trauma indicates a significant burden, probably more than you can resolve on your own, so take action.

---

# LEARN WHAT MAKES YOU HAPPY

Ample evidence shows that negative emotions can suppress immunity and stimulate inflammation (Owen and Steptoe 2003). So how can we be happy? If told it's necessary to be happy for the sake of healing, you might respond, "I just got a cancer diagnosis and you're telling me to be happy?" At the risk of oversimplifying, one of the keys to happiness is finding love in your life: being with people you love and doing what you love, whether it's work or play, and including self-expression, self-nurturing, and a sense of purpose. Good lifestyle habits are essential too, especially right after a stressful event, because it takes *energy* to generate a positive attitude.

Psychotherapist Lawrence LeShan (1999) takes the approach of emphasizing what's right in your life rather than what's wrong. When he began his career, he practiced as he'd been trained: to find out what was wrong with the patient. Though he felt this approach might be useful in some cases, he knew it didn't mobilize the immune system, so he changed his approach by asking patients what would lead them to the greatest enthusiasm and satisfaction in their lives, swhat kind of meaning and purpose would make them glad to get out of bed in the morning and look forward to each day. The psychotherapy process became an exploration of how to create that fulfilled life and move step by step in that direction every day. The goal with this method became to create health rather than fight disease. In this healing context, releasing emotional blockages and processing old traumas became necessary to allow patients to find their own personal individual "songs" and be able to sing them.

# CHAPTER 10

# Psychospiritual Healing

*The best and most beautiful things in the world cannot be seen or even touched. They must be felt with the heart.*

—Helen Keller

For centuries people with great minds and hearts—scientists, philosophers, and spiritual leaders—have discussed questions of mortality, spirituality, and the meaning of life. When people have a cancer diagnosis, their thoughts inevitably lead to the certainty of our mortality. Even though you know you won't live in your body forever, being forced to face that fact greatly focuses and expands your thinking beyond the limits of day-to-day life. Some people spend a lifetime spiritually seeking, while others are comfortable with a religion and a fixed set of beliefs. Most of us have room for more healing in this area, which can bring us to a new level of awareness about the purpose of our existence.

# WHAT IS PSYCHOSPIRITUAL HEALING?

Let's start by clarifying some terms and definitions to help formulate a strategy for coming to terms with the most essential part of our existence. In this book *psychospiritual* means the realm of our existence that encompasses mind and spirit.

## What Is Spirit?

The nonphysical aspect of existence, spirit is separate from but interpenetrates the world of matter and energy. In many religious traditions, spirit is thought to be the aspect of existence that's conscious and animates the physical world. Hard-core materialistic science rejects the existence of spirit, except as an emergent property of matter. In the scientific world, information can be considered a fundamental property of the universe outside of, but related to, the world of mass and energy. Atheists and agnostics often don't believe that there's any continuity of consciousness or a soul entity that lives beyond the time of death. Regardless of belief system, the information in this chapter can be useful to anyone, with or without a cancer diagnosis, who's concerned with longevity and quality of life.

## What Is the Mind?

The mind is more than just the activity of the brain and its conscious thought processes. In traditional East Asian cultures, particularly China and Japan, the mind and "heart" are considered as a unity. The Chinese character (Nelson and Haig 1997) for "mind" 心 also means "heart," referring to the physical organ. The word for "thought" combines the character for mind 心 with the character for "sound" or "noise" 音. The implication of the resulting character for thought 意 is clear.

Thought, *yì* (ibid.)

Thought is not the actual mind, but the *sound* of the mind, the noise the mind makes. The constant chatter in our brains is not the mind, only a part of it, with limitations and weaknesses.

New insights recognize three brains in the body: the "cerebral" brain of the central nervous system, the "heart" brain, and the "enteric" brain of the digestive system. Each brain works independently but communicates with the others constantly and intimately. The "mind" is the flow of information among these different brains and is constantly influenced by their interactions with each other and the environment. We're all fairly familiar with the cerebral brain, but let's take a look at two less familiar ideas: the heart brain and the gut brain.

## THE HEART BRAIN

Thousands of nerve cells in the heart are in constant communication with nerve cells of the brain. In the embryo's development, the heart tissue eventually becomes the tissue that makes up the brain (Pearsall 2007). The heart is associated with emotional intelligence: empathy, compassion, enthusiasm, and joyfulness are part of the language of the heart in its normal functioning. The heart's communication with the brain is a new focus of medical research (Penn and Bakken 2007).

An organization called HeartMath is dedicated to developing this concept of unifying heart and mind. The Institute of HeartMath was founded in 1991 to promote "heart-based living," defined as relying on the intelligence of the heart in concert with the mind, and it has created practical tools that have been scientifically developed and tested (www.heartmath.org/for-you/solutions-for-stress.html). Heart rate variability (HRV) is a tool to evaluate stress and the coordination among the different systems of the body. The rhythm of a healthy heart under resting conditions is actually irregular, and such variations in heart rate aren't usually taken into account when heart rate is calculated. The HRV measurement, derived from the electrocardiogram (ECG), measures the naturally occurring changes in heart rate. Thoughts, feelings, movement, and other physical functions influence variations in heart rate, and also reflect creative ability and how the brain processes information. The rate variations also reflect how we feel, and serve as an objective and noninvasive method to measure and evaluate interactions among the mental, emotional, and behavioral processes of the body's brains. Health and well-being are the result of the harmonious coordination of these brains, and can now be measured objectively. The degree of harmony in this method of testing is called *coherence*. Balance of these brains and their rhythms not only indicates good emotional health but also can indicate physical health and even long-term survival (Dekker et al. 1997).

Doctors Antonio and Hanna Damasio founded the Brain and Creativity Institute at the University of Southern California to research the nature of human emotions, decision making, memory, and communication from a neurological perspective. Dr. Antonio Damasio teaches that science has often overlooked emotions as the source of a person's true identity, so as a neuroscientist, he has focused on the importance of emotions, not just on the cognitive aspects of brain function. He has shown that emotions can be identified with patterns of our physiology and has pointed out that consciousness has multiple levels, many of which can't be put into words. These levels of awareness can be measured through changes in the intensity of our bodies' autonomic responses and through neuronal activity in specific parts of the brain (Damasio et al. 2000).

Humor is one of the languages of the heart. Psychologists who've studied humor note that there's sometimes an element of surprise with a joke's punch line and that the skewed logic in humor can short-circuit the cerebral brain (Sahakian and Frishman 2007). There's also often an element of suffering at the core of humor. These characteristics of suffering and nonlinear logic are in the domain of the heart brain. Humor's effects on the physiology are profound, reducing stress hormones and increasing endorphin levels in the brain. The use of humor for healing came to public awareness when noted author Norman Cousins used laughter to recover from a serious illness and documented his experience in *Anatomy of an Illness As Perceived by the Patient* (W. W. Norton and Company, 1979).

### THE ENTERIC BRAIN

More instinctive than the heart brain, the enteric (gut) brain was identified by Dr. Michael Gershon (1998), who observed that many brain neurotransmitters are found in the intestines and that hormones in the digestive system are also found in the brain. The neurotransmitter serotonin, which is so important to normal sleep and mood regulation, was first discovered in the intestine. The gut actually secretes 95 percent of the body's serotonin, which influences the workings of the digestive tract as well as nerves that signal the brain and reside within the brain itself. Dr. Gershon writes (ibid.) that the intestine can be considered a "brain," because it can "go it alone" (3) without taking orders from the brain; for example, it constantly distinguishes between what's "me" and what's "not me," and decides to either assimilate or eliminate substances in its passageways. This selection process also interacts closely with immunity. The gut's chemistry, physiology, and electrical activity are so much like the central nervous system that it can be called "the brain gone south" (175).

This enteric brain is also an important part of the immune system, which also decides what's "me" and what's "not me." We can allow the enteric brain to reset and work in conjunction with the rest of the body when we follow the guidelines of the five-day diet outlined in chapter 4.

# FINDING MEANING

When facing an apparently life-threatening situation, people often turn to God or a religious practice. Even for people without any religious orientation, finding a special meaning in their lives can serve a useful purpose. Asking and discussing the questions "What's my role?" and "What's my purpose?" can have a therapeutic value. Not everyone has a religious orientation, but even confirmed atheists or nihilists might want to consider the sensibilities of the people who love and care for them. In nearly all cases, there's a benefit, even a sense of relief, in discussing death, with the ultimate result of increasing one's strength to come to terms with life. The French existentialist philosophers proposed that we can only come to terms with life when we're willing to face head-on the fact of our eventual death. The search for meaning takes many forms: we can ask, "What's my purpose in life?" "What are my most important goals for the coming year?" "What do I want my life to stand for?" Strictly from a therapeutic viewpoint, the act of engaging in this process has significant rewards in quality of life and even longevity (Laubmeier, Zakowski, and Bair 2004).

## Near-Death Experiences

When confronted with issues of life and death, it's important to realize that life is much bigger than we imagine. Since the 1980s, open-minded religious leaders and scientists alike have studied the phenomenon of near-death experiences. *Near-death experiences* (*NDEs*) occur when someone comes close to death in an accident or during surgery, often with termination of the heartbeat, and then returns to normal consciousness. Most people, however, return to an *enhanced* normal consciousness, losing their fear of death and either experiencing a strengthened religious commitment or developing one when they'd previously had none. These experiences are now known to be more common than previously believed, with as many as one in five patients who had cardiac arrest during surgery reporting having had an NDE (van Lommel et al. 2001). Substantial literature details this subject, including *Life After Life* by Raymond Moody, Jr. (Bantam Books, 1981), *Nothing Better Than Death* by Kevin Williams (Xlibris Corporation, 2002), and *On Life After Death* by Elizabeth Kübler-Ross (Ten Speed Press, 2008). You can also find a list of titles at www.near-death.com.

Despite the variations of NDE experience, there are many recurrent themes that are strikingly similar, regardless of religion or culture. People often sense a deep feeling of peace and believe that they're traveling through a long tunnel toward an indescribably bright light, where they meet departed loved ones or a deeply compassionate and loving spiritual being, who sometimes tells them that their time of death hasn't arrived. People interviewed about their NDEs often express a certainty about the authenticity of the experience. Even years later, they claim that the memory of the NDE is still fresh and doesn't have the vague quality of a dream but is a daily tangible reality that affects how they conduct their lives.

One thing we can gain from learning about NDEs is a greater perspective. When we look at the larger reality or a more expanded picture of the universe, which our mortality ultimately forces us to do, we can form more authentic goals and put the superficial ones in perspective.

# MEDITATION

You can develop a more powerful faith and ability to live in the present using the time-honored practice of meditation. About ten million people meditate every day in the Western world, and probably many more do so in other parts of the world. A variety of meditation techniques are available from assorted teachings, some traditional and some modern. What they have in common is the intention to look inward, by the act of observing thought processes without participating in them or, in some cases, substituting a thought or sound, called a *mantra*, to occupy the mental space normally cluttered with random thoughts. Observing thought processes from "outside" of them separates us from our identification with them. We begin to identify with another aspect of the self, because there has to be an observer observing the thoughts. The observer, staying in the present moment, observing the parade of ideas floating on our brain waves, experiences a greater version of the mind and often a separation from suffering. Why do we hear about the importance of meditation? It's a practice found in religious thought in both the East and West. Because the present moment is truly all that exists, we need to focus our attention on it in order to find peace and understand the true meaning of mindfulness, which is the experience of being engaged solely in the present. When we drift away from the present, we encounter unreality and certain types of pain that are caused by our relationship to time.

**Grief:** Grief is our experience of pain with respect to the past. We grieve our losses, our lost opportunities, and lost loved ones. We grieve the hurtful things we've done to others and the hurtful things they've done to us, carrying a reservoir of grief and sadness over what was done and what might have been.

**Fear:** Fear is our experience of pain with regard to how we see the future. We now face or ultimately will face many significant fears, but above all is fear of the unknown. The nature of the future is its intrinsic quality of being unknown. If we're sick, we also face the fear of suffering. Unless we have a deep spiritual commitment or experience of life, we face the fear of nothingness, the loss of self and life, the loss of who we are. We fear being alone, the fact that we face death alone and that we have to cross this major hurdle of life without a hand to hold. We fear saying good-bye to our loved ones, especially spouses and children. With our children we face confronting our parental instincts to protect them and avoid leaving them behind. We also fear unfinished business, the feeling of loss over goals we set out for ourselves that we haven't accomplished. The best thing we can give our loved ones is the gift of love, to share the most authentic expression of who we are. If there's not "quantity time," real quality time can be worth years of ordinary mundane experience. We may actually live longer if we create a healing environment within ourselves that extends to our surrounding environment, but even if we don't get those extra years, we have the possibility of being truly present in a way that we seldom allow ourselves to be.

**Pain:** The cure for our pain related to the past and future is to learn to live in the present, which is why we meditate. Being in the present, living in the moment and feeling our connection to life, can have powerful healing properties. In a very literal sense, the present moment is all that exists, and it's where we can find a lot of our healing. The past is gone, and the future doesn't exist. We can be reborn into the present, and enforce forgiveness by staying in the present; remaining in the present can play an important role in resolving past issues.

**Changing the Future:** If we believe that we can influence the future, our relationship to it must be a creative one, and the power of visualization shouldn't be underestimated. Many writers and lecturers on how to succeed speak of the power of visualization. The Bible says that faith is the "assurance of things hoped for and the evidence of things unseen." Faith is an act of powerful visualization, not a set of beliefs. Beliefs may vary from denomination to religion to sect, but faith is power.

## Benefits of Meditation

Besides expanding the mind and freeing us from suffering, meditation yields additional benefits, including reduced stress, improved immunity, and an enhancement of the body's ability to heal.

### MEDITATION AND STRESS REDUCTION

Substantial scientific literature shows that meditation can make people healthier and happier, as well as alter brain structure and possibly even lengthen life span. Meditation's stress-reducing benefits have been established for decades, and they appear to increase with practice. Slowing the brain waves to the alpha state, and even slower, is associated with peacefulness and a sense of well-being. The brain waves from different parts of the brain eventually begin to vibrate together in harmony, a beneficial effect that continues outside of meditation sessions into everyday life experience (Lutz et al. 2004).

Studies have shown that even in beginners, meditation slows respiration and heart rate, lowers blood pressure, improves circulation and sleep, decreases anxiety and depression, improves postoperative healing, and reduces chronic pain, among many other benefits (Grossman et al. 2004). Studies have also shown that cancer patients, who often suffer from high levels of stress, benefit from meditation (Carlson et al. 2004).

### MEDITATION AND IMMUNITY

The immune, nervous, and digestive systems, the brain, and the blood cells are all closely connected. According to research in the new field of psychoneuroimmunology (Pert 1999), the immune system constantly exchanges information with the brain. This new branch of science combines knowledge of psychology, neurology, immunology, and other aspects of physiology to learn the scientific connections between the mind and the body. One way meditation can boost immunity is by increasing the activity of NK cells (Witek-Janusek et al. 2008). Meditation may also reduce production of certain pro-inflammatory cytokines by reducing nervous system activity and changing the brain's chemistry. Researchers at Emory University School of Medicine have also proposed mechanisms by which the body may control the inflammatory response with meditation (Pace et al. 2006).

## MEDITATION AND HEALING

Australian veterinarian Ian Gawler embodies how meditation can play a major role in creating a healing miracle. Gawler was at the advanced stages of bone cancer, which had spread throughout his body, causing deformity in the bones of his chest and pelvis. The cancer had eaten so deeply into the tissues that he had to have his right leg amputated. He also had other conventional medical treatments for a year, but nothing stopped the progression of the disease.

With an extremely poor prognosis from this very aggressive form of bone cancer, and at this late stage, Gawler pulled out all the stops to try to heal himself. He developed his own healing regimen of complementary healing practices consisting of intensive meditation (three one-hour sessions a day), relaxation, positive thinking, a strict diet with nutritional supplements, and even psychic surgery. After he'd pursued this for several months, his doctor could see obvious improvement. The cancer was still present, but he was still alive, and his quality of life had improved. After months of this routine of intensive meditation, the bone tumors started to dissolve until they were completely gone!

Today, in 2009, Ian Gawler is still alive and well, and travels, counseling cancer patients on how to find the inner peace for healing (www.gawler.org). He documented his story in a book, *You Can Conquer Cancer: Prevention and Management* (Michelle Anderson Publishing 2005), which explains a whole philosophy of life based on traditional and spiritual teachings from cultures worldwide. His remarkable "spontaneous remission" was reported in the *Medical Journal of Australia* (Meares 1978).

# How to Meditate

There are lots of ways to meditate; some instructors or systems demand a certain type of attention or the use of a prayer, phrase, or mantra as part of the technique, but there are many variations. Some approaches are more relaxed and some more disciplined. It's a matter of choice as to what feels right for you. If you prefer a structured approach, it's probably beneficial to find a teacher or join a group that convenes regularly.

## Types of Meditation to Try

Two main types of meditation have been the subject of numerous studies, Transcendental Meditation, or TM, with research going as far back as the 1970s (Paul-Labrador et al. 2006), and mindfulness meditation, which was popularized by Jon Kabat-Zinn in the form of the mindfulness-based stress reduction (MBSR) program, about 80 percent of which is meditation (Speca et al. 2000).

**MBSR:** Developed at the University of Massachusetts Medical School (UMASS), MBSR is increasingly being adopted by medical centers throughout the United States and has also been approved in the United Kingdom for use with patients suffering from chronic depression. At UMASS Dr. Kabat-Zinn founded and directed the well-respected Stress Reduction Clinic and, later, the Center for Mindfulness in Medicine, Health Care, and Society (www.umassmed.edu/Content.aspx?id=41254&LinkIdentifier=id).

**TM:** The popularity of Transcendental Meditation (TM) grew in the United States in the early 1970s. The subject of more than six hundred scientific studies that validate and measure its physiological benefits, TM is a worldwide organization with training programs available throughout the United States. The technique is simple and brings almost immediate results (www.tm.org).

**Vipassana Meditation:** Claiming ancient roots at the founding of Buddhism, vipassana meditation centers (www.dhamma.org) schedule regular intensive training programs during ten-day silent retreats. *Vipassana* means "to see things as they are." Despite its Buddhist roots, vipassana meditation is a nonsectarian technique that aims at cleansing "mental impurities."

The benefits of practicing meditation in a program offered by an established organization are obvious: the support of committed meditation practitioners and professionals is a resource of limitless value. However, for many people the problem is taking the time and expense. If you have a life-threatening disease and can involve yourself in a practice that's virtually guaranteed to improve quality of life as well as health and longevity, ask yourself how important this is to you, and consider making the commitment.

## Simplified Meditation Practice

In what was called the "Calm Your Stress Study," researchers at Duke University looked for stress-reduction benefits in healthy adults practicing a simplified meditation method. The purpose was to not only simplify the meditation procedure but also remove any unnecessary religious or sectarian connotations to the practice, because some people who could benefit from meditation might object to some of the religious and cultural trappings surrounding some methods. The researchers designed a simple, brief technique that consisted of asking participants to choose a sound, word, or phrase to use as a mantra for their meditation. Participants were then asked to twice daily sit quietly with closed eyes and repeat the mantra for fifteen to twenty minutes, after which they were to sit quietly for a minute or two before resuming normal activities. The participants were trained in four one-hour training sessions and were evaluated for stress monthly for three months. The results clearly showed significant improvement in several stress-related parameters, and such negative emotions as anger, fear, depression, anxiety, hostility, paranoia, and even fatigue dropped by as much as 40 percent from original levels. The study also showed a correlation between improved outcomes and more frequent meditation practice (Lane, Seskevich, and Pieper 2007).

## ULTRASIMPLIFIED MEDITATION PRACTICE

Using the method developed at Duke University for the "Calm Your Stress Study," choose the sound or phrase you'd like to focus on, and start with three minutes of silent meditation. Focus on the *quality* of your experience rather than force yourself to sit restlessly. A good quality experience would be to stay focused on the mantra and let your thoughts drift by without tracking them. Let the quantity of time take care of itself. You may find, as many people have, that you quickly work up to twenty minutes effortlessly. As the length of meditation time increases, the benefits will as well.

*The Tibetan Book of Living and Dying*, by Sogyal Rinpoche (1992), contains helpful guidelines. The author's background is Tibetan Buddhist, but he encourages the reader to find a unique way to meditate and to not get fussy about the rules. Sogyal Rinpoche advocates taking action and seeking a quality experience even if you have to develop your own method. A simple and time-honored procedure for a beginner, without even the need for a mantra, is to "watch" the breath. Simply close your eyes and observe your inhalations and exhalations, paying attention to each one, watching it without trying to control it, and relaxing with each inhalation and exhalation. As little as ten minutes of this practice can create a relaxed sense of well-being and even a mild euphoria. Getting distracted by thoughts doesn't mean that you're doing something wrong. It's like steering an automobile, where you drift slightly to one side or the other and then bring the wheel back to the middle. Noticing that your thoughts are drifting actually shows a heightened awareness that your thoughts have their own momentum and you can separate your attention from them.

## BUT I'M A CHRISTIAN

The foundation for Christian meditation is in the Bible, which mentions meditation twenty times; for example, "His delight is in the law of the Lord, and in his law he meditates day and night" (Psalm 1:2). The Bible instructs followers to think about God's word. In *The Purpose Driven Life* Rick Warren describes meditation as focused thinking. He writes, "Prayer lets you speak to God; meditation lets God speak to you" (2002, 91) and mentions that the Bible promises amazing benefits to followers who meditate.

A form of Christian meditation used by believers for centuries is called the *lectio divina*, which means "sacred reading." Traditionally used in monastic religious orders, it has renewed popularity today. It's a method of internalizing a scripture or teaching first by reading (*lectio*), discursive meditation (*meditation*), affective prayer (*oratio*), and contemplation (*contemplation*). In the first stage, you find a passage and read it deliberately; in the next stage, you reflect on the text; and in the third stage, you talk to God about the reading, asking him to reveal the truth of it; and in the final stage, you internalize the meaning and rest in the divine presence.

The practice of meditation is an integral part of the monastic tradition of prayer, *hesychasm*, "to keep stillness." One example of this practice is the Jesus Prayer, or the Prayer of the Heart, practiced by monks at Mount Athos in Greece, which uses the idea of a mantra in the repetition of the phrase, "Lord Jesus Christ, Son of God, have mercy on me, a sinner," another version of which is "Lord Jesus Christ, have mercy on my soul." This is repeated every waking moment until it's "internalized" as a constant prayer.

For further information on Christian meditation, refer to The World Community for Christian Meditation website at www.wccm.org.

**Integrating Prayer and Meditation:** The line between meditation and prayer is very narrow. If you have religious convictions, prayer may already be a part of your life. Meditation can help you deepen your experience of prayer. If you've read of saints or devoted souls who had a deep spiritual understanding and awakening, you might ask how they achieved this depth of awareness and contemplation. The way to pray at that level is to meditate deeply and pray from the heart center.

How do you pray if you don't have any religious beliefs? Perhaps you don't pray; perhaps you meditate for the sake of its scientifically proven benefits. If you want to attempt something like prayer, meditate on the heart brain, which might not be an experience of the divine but will be an authentic experience of yourself and could perhaps lead to a deeper experience of your selfhood.

## Variations on Meditation Practice

Other ways, outside of traditional practices, are available to pursue meditation. Modern technology offers us techniques like biofeedback and brain wave synchronization. Biofeedback lets us feel our way into the deeper, slower brain wave states by means of visual or auditory cues; for example, we can see a light or hear a sound when in the alpha brain wave state, and learn how to feel our way into that state more easily by noticing that signal when we're on track.

Brain wave synchronization uses earphones to play music that contains hidden sounds or high-frequency sounds that are slightly different in the left and right earphone speakers. The slight difference in frequency causes not necessarily audible beats. These beats can be set to vibrate at the alpha wave frequency (eight to twelve beats per second), for example, and gradually create "entrainment" from the listener's brain waves to that frequency.

Another variation of meditation practice is visualization. Visualization techniques are popularly taught to help people program their minds toward success, but some have been designed specifically for healing. One method that has actually been researched and used with cancer patients is that of Dr. O. Carl Simonton, described in his book *Getting Well Again* (Simonton, Matthews-Simonton, and Creighton 1992; available at www.simontoncenter.com). In this method, you visualize your white blood cells (especially NK cells) destroying the cancer in your body. Imagine that a very active swarm of white blood cells scintillates with vitality and attaches itself to toxic cells, tumor fragments, and toxic microbes, causing them to explode. You can then visualize the bloblike macrophages gobbling up the residue. Many people have created their own variations of this visualization, and research results have shown a favorable response with patients who practice this (Simonton, Matthews-Simonton, and Sparks 1980).

## *Healing Through Service and Self-Expression*

G. J. was diagnosed with malignant melanoma at age forty. Though she had it surgically removed, because her father and his four sisters had all died of cancer, she found herself in a state of abject terror. She'd been an art student before working as a circuit-board designer in an electronics company, and later found that painting brought her deep satisfaction. She didn't adopt a special diet or any supplements until much later but quit her job and moved to the country. Still consumed with fear of death and dying, she consulted a Native American healer, who recommended that she work with dying people. She began to visit nursing homes and was inspired by many people who, although frail, possessed strong, vibrant spirits. She made paintings for them and let these experiences open her heart and help her let go of the fear of cancer and its recurrence. Now, twenty-five years later, she says that she has no special rules; she eats intuitively and feels that a lot of "static" has been removed so that she can feel "higher frequencies."

# Moving Meditation: Yoga, Tai Chi, Qigong, and Other Martial Arts

As mentioned in chapter 8, several East Asian methods have gained widespread popularity in Western culture since the 1960s. Yoga exists in many forms, but the best known is hatha yoga, which uses various body postures to stretch out the muscles, relieve tension, and create a calm condition conducive to the meditative state. As you've learned, tai chi and qigong are forms of moving meditation. A type of dance, tai chi is also the foundation for many movements used in martial arts. Both tai chi and qigong coordinate movement with the breath to achieve coherence, or mind-body harmonization. Qigong is a type of breathing in and out of the life force, known as *qi* in Chinese. The word "qi" has nuances related to air and the breath, similar to the Sanskrit word "prana" or the Greek "pneuma," both of which also imply a relation of vital force to the breath and the ability to control it.

Martial arts can be a useful healing tool. Many martial arts masters specialize in using the arts to cultivate personal harmony, physical and mental strength, and integrity. Whether or not you're the fighter "type," the warrior's path is about the courage to overcome fear.

## The Vision Quest

A vision quest is a retreat for prayer or meditation or for enhancing an inward practice. Most people who go on a vision quest go to connect with nature and with the inner self. The purpose is to strip away the superficial preoccupations with mundane life and search our inner being for what our inner self needs or wants to express. The most famous vision quest was when Jesus fasted for forty days and nights on the mountaintop, where he endured temptation. Whether literal or allegorical forces are encountered, on a vision quest we seek to not only have a peak experience but also discover the dark forces that motivate our lives.

A vision quest can be self-designed; for example, a fishing trip or wilderness hike could set the stage for a successful vision quest. One key element is solitude, and another is communion with nature. In traditional forms, especially in tribal cultures, austerities such as fasting and vigils are an integral part of the experience. But once again, there are as many ways to carry out a vision quest as there are people, as long as it's done with the right spirit and intention. Supervised vision quests and survival training experiences are also available.

---

# ASSESS YOUR LEVEL OF PSYCHOSPIRITUAL CONTENTMENT

Circle "Y" for yes or "N" for no, and mark in one point for each yes answer:

Y or N   _____   Do you enjoy your work?

Y or N   _____   Do you take any time for relaxation?

Y or N   _____   Are you contented in your personal relationships?

Y or N   _____   Do you have a religious belief or practice?

_____   How much time do you spend in inwardly focused activity (such as meditation, prayer, or devotional services)? (one point for more than two hours a week)

If you scored two points, you probably don't need to focus on improving your psychospiritual contentment unless a medical diagnosis has thrown you into an existential crisis. If so, get help. Some support groups have both a spiritual and psychological orientation.

# CHAPTER 11

# Symptom Relief

This chapter focuses on the needs of patients undergoing conventional cancer treatments, such as chemotherapy, radiation, and surgery, whose symptoms can be severe in some cases. Many patients quit treatment because of the severity of symptoms. Usually, if your oncologist doesn't support use of supplements and natural therapies, the main objections are using supplements during the actual course of treatment. At the same time, oncologists often express disinterest in what you eat as long as it's "a good diet." In between courses of treatment, you'll likely be able to use detoxification principles, diet recommendations, and supplements to recover for the next course. Many of the supplements recommended in chapter 6 are actually foods, even if in the form of capsules, tablets, or individually wrapped doses of powders, which is true of AHCC (mushrooms in rice bran), proteolytic enzymes (pineapple and papaya enzymes with sheep pancreas), Avemar (cultured wheat germ), and many of the others.

The most important symptom to deal with, common to all three conventional therapies but especially chemotherapy, is nausea and vomiting, which is usually divided into two categories: early and late. While drugs are often successful at controlling the early nausea, later nausea can be more difficult to control.

## NAUSEA AND VOMITING

There are at least two causes of nausea and vomiting: *mucositis*, which is inflammation of the mucous membranes lining the digestive tract, and signals from the nervous system. In the latter case, nerve signals from the upper part of the small intestine go to the brain and trigger a nausea response. There are many things to try, but first, heed this general advice:

> Eat small, frequent meals during the day.

> To avoid diluting digestive juices, don't drink liquids with food.

> Avoid heavy, oily foods, opting instead for steamed vegetables, fresh fruits, light grains, and proteins.

> Avoid food smells; leave the house when food is being cooked.

> You might want to avoid your favorite foods so that you don't start to associate them with nausea and vomiting.

> Avoid protein foods after 6:00 p.m.

> Avoid sugar; if you need a sweetener, use rice or barley malt, agave nectar, or stevia extract.

> Drink liquids between meals. Preferred temperature is very individual in that some people can only tolerate room temperature, while others prefer ice cold or warm. You decide.

> Rest after eating, but prop up; don't lie flat.

> Smoking will aggravate nausea and vomiting, so it's a good time to quit; consider it one of the benefits of treatment.

> Though habitual smoking of cannabis has been determined to increase the risk of lung cancer, some doctors recommend it for short-term use to counteract the nausea symptoms that often accompany chemotherapy (Machado Rocha et al. 2008). Consider using it if your doctor recommends it and it's from an uncontaminated source, particularly free of fungal growth.

Call your doctor if your nausea completely interferes with your ability to eat; if you're not responding to any antinausea medication or remedy, or are suffering from side effects of the drugs; or if you vomit four to five times in a twenty-four-hour period or feel pain and bloating in the upper abdominal region.

Some treatments using herbs or supplements presuppose that you'll be able to swallow them in pill or capsule form because nausea is under control. As a rule, it's best to avoid alcohol, so you'll want to minimize tincture use except for something like gentian extract (discussed in the next section), whose dose is only one to five drops.

# Very Safe Potential Treatments for Nausea and Vomiting

**Ginger:** Studied for many types of nausea, ginger may help; try it as a tea rather than a tincture or a capsule (Bone et al. 1990). Protein foods with ginger have been studied recently for the difficult-to-treat late-stage nausea, so this might be a better strategy for a lot of people. When it didn't give complete relief, it helped reduce the amount of antinausea medication (Levine et al. 2006).

**DGL** (deglycyrrhizinated licorice): DGL is essentially licorice from which the component "glycyrrhizin" has been removed to help very sensitive stomachs tolerate it. Used to treat stomach ulcers, DGL can help soothe the mucous-membrane inflammation that causes a lot of the discomfort (Morgan et al. 1982).

**Kuzu** (*Pueraria lobata*): Very soothing and also nourishing, kuzu (Japanese arrowroot) resembles little white rocks. Dissolve it in *cold* water, and then heat and simmer it until it thickens and turns clear. Allow it to cool and then drink it. In Japan they often add a little grated ginger on top.

**Clove Oil:** Available at any pharmacy, clove oil can be diluted with just a drop in some water to drink. Repeat if it helps. Allspice, which, like clove, contains eugenol, is another herb that has been used for chemotherapy nausea. Eugenol is the active principle that causes local numbness and is used by dentists to swab inside the mouth to numb the site of injection. Eugenol also has antibacterial (Li et al. 2005) and antifungal (Chami et al. 2005) properties.

**Chamomile:** A very good sedative, chamomile tea works well for stomach upset and to calm the nerves.

**Swedish Bitters:** Swedish bitters is a traditional herbal formula used for digestive and other symptoms that has been helpful to some people with nausea and vomiting; use a very small dose at first to see how well you tolerate it.

**Gentian:** Available in a tincture, gentian is a classic bitter digestive herb. Just one drop can make a difference. Despite its bitterness, many people suffering from nausea find the flavor pleasant. If it works for you, as little as five drops is enough for an effective dose.

**Slippery Elm:** Very soothing to the mucous membranes, slippery elm is also traditionally used for stomach ulcers. If you're very sensitive, just chew on the dried herb to get relief.

**Acupressure:** Some people find nausea relief from pressing an acupuncture point known as the antinausea point. You can find it by turning your palm upward and placing three fingers from your other hand on the wrist crease perpendicularly. The distance three perpendicular fingers up from the wrist crease, toward the middle of the (palmar) forearm, is the point where you apply gentle pressure. You can do this on either the left or right arm. You'll probably find that one side is more tender than the other, and that side is often more effective at relieving nausea.

# SYMPTOMS OF DEHYDRATION

Dehydration can result from vomiting, diarrhea, or both. Its symptoms are decreased urine output; dark urine; dry mouth, skin, and lips; a dry appearance to the eyeballs; difficulty swallowing; confusion; dizziness, especially when standing up; rapid, pounding, or irregular heartbeat; and even fainting. The obvious cure is to drink water, but if you can't even keep water down, try holding an ice chip in your mouth. Try taking small amounts of water, just a couple of small swallows, every fifteen minutes. Reverse-osmosis-filtered water or distilled water has a better chance of being absorbed before coming back up. If you can keep fluids down, sports electrolyte drinks can speed up rehydration. If dehydration persists, consider trying to get fluid intravenously at your doctor's office or a hospital.

If you've been vomiting, it's necessary to prevent dehydration and loss of electrolytes. Try Emergen-C as first aid, but vegetable stocks made with added sea salt, or miso broth using a seaweed or fish stock is best of all. As a reminder, miso is a salty paste from Japan made from soybeans cultured in sea salt. Rich in friendly bacteria, electrolytes, and enzymes, it should be stirred into hot water but never boiled. Truly one of the world's great healing foods, miso is very warming, nourishing, and healing.

# ACID REFLUX

Acid reflux is when acid from the stomach rises up the esophagus, often causing a burning sensation. In some cases you can treat acid reflux with alkalizers to neutralize or reduce excess acidity. Plant anti-inflammatories useful for reflux include noni juice, which is from a tropical fruit rich in the anti-inflammatory enzyme bromelain. Available in spray bottles, vitamin U is actually an extract from an African plant in the cabbage family that may help with acid reflux. You can also benefit from juicing cabbages (Cheney 1949). Cabbage juice is traditionally used in Europe as a remedy for stomach ulcers. Swedish bitters can also help with acid reflux.

# CONSTIPATION

If you're constipated, are you drinking enough water? Drink water in smaller quantities more frequently, and make sure you eat enough fruit and fiber. Prune juice actually works for a lot of people's constipation. Use strong laxatives like senna or cascara sagrada cautiously. However, taking pure aloe in tablets is safe to experiment with, because aloe is also known to boost immunity. Psyllium husks bulk the stool, but ground flaxseeds are even better, because they contain lignans that protect against cancer (Thompson et al. 2005). Flaxseeds are also a source of omega-3 fatty acids. Grind and add them to a shake. Acupuncturists and ayurvedic practitioners often provide gentle herbal formulas for chronic constipation. You might also try commercial preparations, such as Fleet Enema or glycerine suppositories. Call your doctor if severe or persistent abdominal pain, swelling, or increased nausea and vomiting accompany your constipation.

# DIARRHEA

Chemotherapy can cause diarrhea, but so can radiation treatment or surgery, especially to the abdominal area, and even bone-marrow transplants. Some types of cancer also cause diarrhea, especially colon, pancreatic, liver, and gallbladder cancers; and lymphoma. Call your doctor if diarrhea persists and you're suffering from dehydration, or if you have black or bloody stools, fever, or severe or persistent cramps. Possible causes are anxiety and stress, antibiotics, and food intolerances, such as to dairy products. You might have intolerances while undergoing medical treatment that you don't have otherwise. Foods sweetened with sorbitol can cause diarrhea. Avoid heavy, greasy and fried foods, and raw foods in favor of bland, cooked foods, including proteins. Bananas can sometimes slow down diarrhea, and carob powder can help. Another folk remedy is boiled sweet potatoes or boiled blueberries. Lactobacillus acidophilus can relieve diarrhea and restore the healthful bacteria in the digestive tract. Foods that are low in fiber, such as white rice and vegetables, which are high in potassium, can prevent irritation. Several over-the-counter remedies are available at pharmacies, but herbalists, including acupuncturists and ayurvedic practitioners, offer safe and effective remedies.

# ALTERNATING CONSTIPATION AND DIARRHEA

If you have alternating constipation and diarrhea, discuss this with your doctor or other health care provider. Acupuncturists, ayurvedic practitioners, and nutritionists often have safe and specific treatments for this confounding problem.

# POOR DIGESTION

*Acidophilus bifidus* and *Saccharomyces boulardii* are probiotic preparations containing healthful microbes that can relieve most digestive symptoms as well as improve digestive efficiency. The amino acid glutamine nourishes the digestive tract and also helps with sugar cravings. Digestive enzymes can also help get digestion back on track and also relieve symptoms of overeating.

# SORE MOUTH AND THROAT (FROM MUCOSITIS)

A common symptom from chemotherapy or radiation to the head and neck area is sore mouth or throat from mucositis, which often occurs three to seven days after treatment. Sometimes sores and ulcerations form in the mouth. Mucositis in the digestive tract also possibly causes some of the hypersensitivity that results in discomfort from nausea, constipation, and diarrhea. Taking vitamin E (mixed tocopherol) with chemotherapy can improve treatment response and prevent mucositis (Ferreira et al. 2004). In a study at the Veterans Administration Medical Center in Washington, D.C., vitamin E oil (400 IU per cubic centimeter) was rubbed into the skin around the neck, and still prevented inflammation and ulcer formation (Wadleigh et al. 1992). The medical treatment for such symptoms is usually steroids, which can worsen stomach sensitivity and lower immunity.

# HAIR LOSS (ALOPECIA)

If you have hair loss, ask your doctor if a *cold cap* procedure is available. A cold cap is a type of headgear that cools the scalp for a period before and after chemotherapy. Cooling the scalp restricts blood circulation to the hair follicles to restrict the amount of the chemotherapy drug that reaches the scalp. The type of cold cap used varies from one clinic to the next. The cap is usually put on fifteen minutes before chemotherapy and worn during it, as well as for one to two hours after the chemotherapy session. The cold caps are effective in preventing hair loss for most chemotherapy drugs (Grevelman and Breed 2005). One observation reported in the *New England Journal of Medicine* showed the potential for vitamin E to prevent hair loss from chemotherapy (Wood 1985). As I learned while living in Japan, clinicians there have observed that some patients taking AHCC don't lose their hair from cancer treatment.

# WEIGHT LOSS AND MALNUTRITION (CACHEXIA)

Cachexia is more than just weight loss; it's a severe weakening and wasting away that's responsible for 20 percent of cancer deaths (Muscaritoli et al. 2006). The condition is the result of breakdown, not only of fatty tissue but also muscles and even the smooth muscle that makes up organs and their membranes. Hydrazine sulfate has been used for cachexia for over thirty years, but its use is controversial in the United States. Several studies in the United States showed no results, although some showed improved quality of life (National Cancer Institute 2008). Critics of the negative U.S. studies stated that it's ineffective if used with tranquilizers, barbiturates, or alcohol and that 94 percent of the patients in the negative studies used at least one of these. Hydrazine sulfate is used in Europe, Canada, and Russia with a response rate between 60 and 70 percent (Filov et al. 1995). Some studies, including one in the United States, even showed some degree of tumor reduction (Chlebowski et al. 1990). Hydrazine sulfate is a MAO inhibitor (a substance that inhibits the destruction of brain neurotransmitters called *monoamines*, such as dopamine and noradrenalin; MAO inhibitor drugs require patients who take them to observe a strict diet to prevent side effects or inactivation), so there are several other foods and substances that can inactivate it: antihistamines, opiates, foods containing tyramine (red wine, some types of cheese, and several other food items), and vitamins B6 and C. It's also useful to take very concentrated foods like fruit juice (such as mangosteen or pomegranate) with other nutrients or include them in a shake to more easily absorb the nutrients. Don't use hydrazine without first consulting a qualified health care practitioner.

# WEAKNESS AND FATIGUE

Juice fasting can energize you and speed up your recovery from cancer treatment, unless you're suffering severe weight loss (see the recovery protocol at the end of this chapter). Exercise is also necessary to help with weakness and fatigue. Ginseng is a well-tested remedy for increasing stamina in weakened patients. Another Chinese herb, astragalus, can also help. $CoQ_{10}$ can provide a noticeably energizing effect in a short time. Use at least 60 milligrams a day for this purpose. Hydrolyzed whey protein dissolved in rice, hemp, or nut milk (but not soy milk) can boost energy, and vitamin E (succinate or mixed tocopherols) can also help.

# LOSS OF LIBIDO

Fortunately, low libido usually clears up after the course of treatment. Ginseng and other traditional Chinese and ayurvedic herbs can sometimes make a difference. Research shows that increased exercise can help improve sexual function (Penedo and Dahn 2005). Kegel exercises, which strengthen the groin muscles, can also help some aspects of sexual dysfunction. Levels of the hormone DHEA are low in both men and women with sexual dysfunction, but neither DHEA nor testosterone supplementation is recommended for use by people with breast, endometrial, or prostate cancer (Kaaks et al. 2005). DHEA is also not recommended for liver cancer patients. Education about sexual function has helped some patients, and acupuncture and massage for stress reduction can improve well-being and support restoring libido.

# LOW IMMUNITY

Chemotherapy and radiation are responsible for negative effects on the bone marrow, blood, and lymph, resulting in lowered immunity. The risk of infection is a life-threatening hazard in patients with damaged immunity from chemotherapy or radiation. Here are some helpful supplements:

**AHCC:** Helps with numerous chemotherapy side effects; increases NK cell activity; prevents leukopenia (reduced white blood cell count) and anemia; and protects the bone marrow, and therefore red and white blood cell production (Won 2002) (see chapter 6).

**Alkylglycerols:** Fatty substances, also called *ether lipids*, that are usually derived from shark liver oil (but be sure they're free of PCBs) but are also found in human milk (less so in cow's milk). Alkylglycerols support bone marrow function, and prevent low red cell count (anemia) and low platelet count (thrombocytopenia) (Pugliese et al. 1998).

**Ashwagandha:** Ayurvedic herb that can protect bone marrow and prevent low platelet count (Davis and Kuttan 1998).

**Avemar:** Prevents leukopenia (low white cell count), exposes hidden cancer cells to destruction by the immune system (see chapter 6).

**Astragalus:** Prevents leukopenia (see chapter 6).

**Hydrolyzed whey protein:** Helps with anemia and fatigue, and stimulates glutathione (the detoxifying amino acid) production.

**Liver extract:** Liquid liver and desiccated liver extracts can treat anemia, raising red blood cell count.

**Vitamin B12:** Treats anemia and works well with folate; ask your doctor about the possibility of supplementing with folate during chemotherapy, and about getting B12 injections. Anemia is a common side effect of cancer treatment, and using B12 and folate as supplements can help even if blood tests show normal levels (Naurath et al. 1995).

**Vitamin E:** Can protect bone marrow (vitamin E succinate) (see chapter 6).

**Selenium:** Can protect white blood cells from chemotherapy (Asfour et al. 2006).

The following supplements are particularly helpful for these blood-related symptoms:

> ➤ Anemia (low red cell count): Liver extracts, vitamin B12, folate, alkylglycerols, hydrolyzed whey protein

> Leukopenia (low white cell count): AHCC, astragalus, Avemar, ginseng (American, Chinese, or Siberian), echinacea, ashwagandha, alkylglycerols, viamin E, vitamin C, zinc, selenium, glutamine (2 to 4 grams a day)

> Myelosuppression (bone marrow suppression): AHCC, alkylglycerols, vitamin E

> Thrombocytopenia (low platelet count): Alkylglycerols, ashwagandha

# NERVOUS SYSTEM SYMPTOMS

**Anxiety and Depression:** If you don't want to use a prescription drug for anxiety and depression, a lot of options are available. Don't underrate talk therapy. If you feel that your problem is serious, talk to a professional, but sharing your feelings with a confidant can also be extremely helpful. Though St. John's wort is often mentioned for depression, it can be mildly stimulating and thus may not be appropriate for anxiety along with depression. It's also photosensitizing, so if you take it, cover up when you're in the sun. A lot of herbal sedatives can be surprisingly helpful, such as skullcap, passionflower, chamomile, and essential oils like lavender. Lithium orotate is not a prescription drug but *nutritional* lithium, which we need for brain health. This supplement can help restore normal moods, but be sure to consult a knowledgeable health care provider before experimenting with it. Also be sure to get enough exercise, which stimulates your endorphins (the brain's pleasure chemicals) during that second wind. Stress reduction methods, such as aromatherapy, massage, and acupuncture also get your endorphins flowing again.

**Headache:** I recommend magnesium orotate or aspartate for headaches and spasms. Oil of peppermint or peppermint blended with rosemary rubbed on the neck and shoulders can give surprising relief.

**Insomnia:** The amino acids 5-HTP, found in the herb griffonia (*Griffonia simplicifolia*), and tryptophan can relieve insomnia. Herbs like valerian, chamomile, skullcap, and passionflower can provide deeper sleep. Aromatherapy, massage, acupuncture, or any other stress reduction will help if you're committed to a more relaxed lifestyle.

**Peripheral Neuropathy:** Alpha-lipoic acid (200 to 600 milligrams a day), acupuncture, and vitamin E (600 IU a day) can prevent neuropathy in some chemotherapy patients (Argyriou et al. 2005). Omega-3 fatty acids from fish oil or other sources are also protective. Phosphatidylcholine, found in lecithin, helps protect nerve membranes. B vitamins, especially B6 and B12, are useful for neuropathy.

**Cognitive Decline ("Chemobrain" or "Brain Fog"):** The "smart drug" Provigil (modafinil) improved cognitive function in breast-cancer chemotherapy patients (Whyche 2007). Alcohol and sugar greatly aggravate this symptom. Ginseng (1,000 to 2,000 milligrams a day) is known to protect nerve tissue (Barton et al. 2007), and alpha-lipoic acid slows down age-related cognitive decline and thus might be useful, since it's a powerful antioxidant (200 to 600 milligrams a day) (Hager et al. 2001).

# CARDIOVASCULAR SYMPTOMS

Evidence shows that vitamin E could prevent heart damage (Nandave et al. 2007). Though inconclusive in human trials, there's evidence that vitamin E enhances treatment effects and improves tolerance of Adriamycin (doxorubicin) (Puri et al. 2001). Studies with both animals and humans have found that pretreating with $CoQ_{10}$, at levels of 100 milligrams a day, reduces cardiac toxicity caused by Adriamycin (Judy et al. 1984). I recommend the liquid form of CoQ10 at a higher dose, around 200 to 300 milligrams a day, which is expensive but important for certain chemotherapy drugs or radiation for the chest or neck area. Taurine (1,000 to 2,000 milligrams a day) also protects the cardiovascular system. Be sure to consult your doctor before taking these supplements.

# SKIN PAIN AND BLISTERS (PALMAR-PLANTAR ERYTHRODYSESTHESIA)

*Palmar-plantar erythrodysesthesia* is pain, blisters, sores, and pigment changes in the hands and feet. A daily dose of vitamin E (450 IU a day), either during or after chemotherapy, caused the lesions and discomfort to disappear after a week in patients receiving radiotherapy (Kara, Sahin, and Erkisi 2006). Topical DMSO (dimethyl sulfoxide) (about twelve drops, four times a day) can also relieve the condition in one to three weeks (Lopez et al. 1999).

# POSTSURGICAL RECOVERY

During recovery from surgery, proteolytic enzymes are helpful for relieving inflammation (Tassman, Zafran, and Zayon 1964), preventing adhesions and scar tissue, and possibly preventing or slowing down metastasis (Cohen et al. 1999). Large doses are necessary for the first few days after surgery. Taking as much as 1,000 milligrams of bromelain (pineapple enzyme), 1,200 milligrams of papain (papaya enzyme), and 2,000 milligrams of pancreatin an hour before or after any food, two to five times a day, for the first three to four days, depending on the size of the surgical wound, and tapering down thereafter should noticeably reduce swelling (Vinzenz 1991).

# THE ROLE OF ACUPUNCTURE

Acupuncture, as well as treatment from a professional massage therapist or structural body-worker, can benefit many of the symptoms in this chapter, particularly any that could be stress related. Acupuncture can help with chemotherapy-related nausea. Acupuncture, ginger, and guided imagery, the subject of numerous studies (Streitberger, Ezzo, and Schneider 2006), are used for chemotherapy-related nausea at the Cleveland Clinic (http://my.clevelandclinic.org). Acupuncture also helps relieve hot flashes, fatigue, and night sweats after breast cancer chemotherapy (Walker et al. 2008). Evidence-based guidelines from the American College of Chest Physicians recommend acupuncture for lung cancer patients who suffer from a variety of symptoms, including fatigue, neuropathy, cognitive decline, nausea, vomiting, and difficulty breathing (Cassileth et al. 2007). Doctors at Duke University concluded that postoperative pain is significantly improved if acupuncture is performed both before and after surgery (Sun et al. 2008). Other research at Duke has evaluated acupuncture as beneficial for headaches, nausea, and sports performance. The most reliable benefit of acupuncture is stress reduction, whose results are cumulative with regular treatment.

# BASIC TREATMENT RECOVERY PROTOCOL

**Decompress Stress:** Get massage, acupuncture, aromatherapy, or just play golf.

**Juice It Up:** Take a day for a juice cleanse. Start out with açaí juice, pomegranate juice, or a blend in the morning. If these aren't easily available, just use cranberry juice or diluted lemon juice. Have several vegetable juices during the day, whenever you feel hungry. It's best to juice the foods freshly, so if you don't have a juicer, plan to borrow one for a few days. I recommend carrot-celery-apple (just a little green apple, pippin, or Granny Smith) or cabbage-celery-romaine-apple juice. Hearty greens like kale are a good addition, and a little watercress, parsley, or ginger will also add some bite. Some people like to use wheatgrass or green barley. You can make up your own formula. Have papaya juice sometime during the day, if you're still queasy from treatment. Have warm, relaxing herbal tea, like chamomile, near bedtime. If you'd like some miso soup, you can have it anytime.

**Five-Day Diet:** Start out by trying the five-day diet recommendations for a day or two. Plan your meals in advance so you'll know what to have when you get hungry. Add protein to any shakes you make. Use rice milk, nut milk, or hemp milk; or add a nutritional blend like UltraClear or PaleoMeal. Work with a nutrition-oriented practitioner to figure out the best ingredients for your particular situation. Have a shake once or twice a day, depending on how hungry you are. Supplement with freshly juiced vegetables. If you're really tired, hydrolyzed whey protein can build up red blood cells and energy, but proceed with caution if you have a dairy allergy. However, sometimes people who are allergic to dairy tolerate it well.

**Supplements:** You might want to discuss with your health care provider the possibility of using some of the detoxifying supplements mentioned in chapter 6.

---

# YOUR SYMPTOMS

List any symptoms you feel you need to focus on:

_____

_____

_____

_____

_____

---

# ISSUES TO DISCUSS WITH YOUR HEALTH CARE PROVIDER

List any questions or issues you want to discuss with one of your health care providers after reviewing the information in this book:

_____

_____

_____

_____

_____

# APPENDIX

# Resources

---

# WEBSITES

For updates on information in this book and for more information on cancer survival tools, go to www.dankennerresearch.com.

## Mainstream Information

American Cancer Society: www.cancer.org

National Cancer Institute: www.cancer.gov or www.nci.nih.gov

Breastcancer.org: www.breastcancer.org

Cancer Survivors Network: http://csn.cancer.org

CancerCare: www.cancercare.org

Association of Cancer Online Resources (information and support groups): www.acor.org

CancerIndex (guide to Internet resources): www.cancerindex.org

## Information on Complementary Approaches

Commonweal (cancer recovery retreats): www.commonweal.org

The Moss Reports (information on complementary cancer treatments): www.ralphmoss.com

Natural Medicines Comprehensive Database: www.naturaldatabase.com

Pine Street Foundation (cancer screening by breath analysis): pinestreetfoundation.org

# BOOKS

Béliveau, R., and D. Gingras. 2006. *Foods That Fight Cancer: Preventing Cancer Through Diet*. Toronto, Canada: McClelland and Stewart.

Bishop, B. 1999. *A Time to Heal: Triumph over Cancer, the Therapy of the Future*. New York: Penguin Arkana.

Boik, J. 2001. *Natural Compounds in Cancer Therapy: Promising Nontoxic Antitumor Agents from Plants and Other Natural Sources*. Princeton, MN: Oregon Medical Press.

Gawler, I. 1987. *You Can Conquer Cancer: Prevention and Management*. London: Thorsons.

Hopko, D., and C. Lejuez. 2007. *A Cancer Patient's Guide to Overcoming Depression and Anxiety: Getting Through Treatment and Getting Back to Your Life*. Oakland, CA: New Harbinger Publications.

## Books by Doctors Who Recovered from Cancer Using Natural Medicine

Blaylock, R. L. 2003. *Natural Strategies for Cancer Patients*. New York: Twin Streams Books.

Sattilaro, A. J. 1982. *Recalled by Life: The Story of My Recovery from Cancer*. Boston: Houghton Mifflin.

Servan-Schreiber, D. 2008. *Anticancer: A New Way of Life*. New York: Viking.

# SUPPLEMENTS

AHCC (active hexose correlated compound): www.ormedinstitute.com, www.ambiosciences.com, www.yesahcc.com

Alkabase (an alkalizer that can be used with proteolytic enzymes or as an antacid): www.ormedinstitute.com

Ashwagandha (*Withania Somnifera*): www.ayurvedicherbsdirect.com

Astragalus: www.chineseherbsdirect.com

Avemar: www.ambiosciences.com

Coenzyme $Q_{10}$ and Ubiquinol (liquid form): www.iherb.com

DGL (deglycyrrhizinated licorice): www.iherb.com, www.bodyandfitness.com

DMSO (dimethyl sulfoxide): Many natural food stores

Electrolyte products: Use alkalizers, sea vegetable extracts (like laminaria), or blue-green algae

Enzymes: See proteolytic enzymes

Essential oils (pharmaceutical grade): www.ormedinstitute.com (peppermint and clove oils available over the counter at most pharmacies)

Garlic products Kyolic from Wakunaga: 800-825-7888 or www.kyolic.com

Ginseng: www.ormedinstitute.com (blend), www.chineseherbsdirect.com

Hydrazine sulphate: www.nextag.com

Laminaria extract (kombu sea vegetable): www.ormedinstitute.com

Modified citrus pectin: Many natural food stores

MSM (methylsulfonylmethane): Many natural food stores

Phosphatidylcholine: www.phoschol.com

Proteolytic enzymes: www.ormedinstitute.com (used primarily for inflammation). Some natural cancer therapies use enzymes especially developed for tumor reduction. They're safe but expensive. Tumor reduction and leukemia formulas are available from College Health Stores, LLC, 410 Lution Drive Weatherford, TX 76087; 888-477-3618. Enzymes should be taken with an alkalizer.

Recancostat (contains detoxifying amino acids and antioxidants from plant sources): Integrative Therapeutics, Inc., 800-380-1819, www.integrativeinc.com

Vitamin U: store.uniflora.us/index.html

# FOODS

Alkylglycerols (shark liver oil): www.cancerchoices.com (differs from shark cartilage, which claims to prevent angiogenesis)

Grass-fed beef: Check for local sources first. I found seven sources just in Northern California:

> Texas: Slanker's www.texasgrassfedbeef.com

> Colorado: Lasater www.lasatergrasslandsbeef.com

> Pennsylvania: www.allnaturalbeefco.com

> Washington: Eatwild (not just beef) www.eatwild.com

Hydrolyzed whey protein: www.imuplus.com

# OTHER RESOURCES

HeartMath (www.heartmath.com): Stress reduction strategies

Wise Brain (www.wisebrain.org): Meditation and brain functioning tools

Tissue mineral analysis (www.ormedinstitute.com): Tests hair sample for heavy metals

PCA3 Test: Though San Diego–based Gen-Probe developed this prostate cancer urine test, it's only available in Europe, as of this book's publication, not in the United States.

HIFU (high-intensity focused ultrasound) (www.hifu.ca or www.internationalhifu.com): Nonsurgical prostate cancer treatment

EDR (extreme drug resistance) testing (www.exiqon.com/dx): Testing for potential effectiveness of chemotherapy

Oncotype DX (www.oncotypedx.com): Testing for potential effectiveness of chemotherapy (Genomic Health, Redwood City, CA)

Reverse-osmosis water filters (www.reverse-osmosis-water-filter-guide.com): Home water-filter systems

Shower filters (www.showerfiltercomparisons.com): Home shower-filters

Infrared saunas: Available at High Tech Health, Boulder, CO (www.hightechhealth.com) and Clearlight (www.infraredsauna.com), but shop around, and if you decide to build your own, be sure to let the formaldehyde off-gas from any wood panels used in construction.

# References

Adam, K., and I. Oswald. 1983. Protein synthesis, bodily renewal, and the sleep-wake cycle. *Clinical Science* 65 (6):561–67.

Ader, R., D. L. Felton, and N. Cohen, eds. 2000. *Psychoneuroimmunology.* 3rd ed. San Diego, CA: Academic Press.

Aggarwal, B. B., A. Kumar, and A. C. Bharti. 2003. Anticancer potential of curcumin: Preclinical and clinical studies. *Anticancer Research* 23 (1A):363–98.

Ahuja, J. K. C., J. D. Goldman, and A. J. Moshfegh. 2004. Current status of vitamin E nutriture. *Annals of the New York Academy of Sciences* 1031:387–90.

Ailhaud, G., and P. Guesnet. 2004. Fatty acid composition of fats is an early determinant of childhood obesity: A short review and an opinion. *Obesity Reviews* 5 (1):21–26.

Ainsworth, B. E., W. L. Haskell, M. C. Whitt, M. L. Irwin, A. M. Swartz, S. J. Strath, W. L. O'Brien, D. R. Bassett Jr., K. H. Schmitz, P. O. Emplaincourt, D. R. Jacobs Jr., and A. S. Leon. 2000. Compendium of physical activities: An update of activity codes and MET intensities. *Medicine and Science in Sports and Exercise* 32 (Suppl. 9):S498–516.

Allen, N. E., C. Sauvaget, A. W. Roddam, P. Appleby, J. Nagano, G. Suzuki, T. J. Key, and K. Koyama. 2004. A prospective study of diet and prostate cancer in Japanese men. *Cancer Causes and Control* 15 (9):911–20.

American Academy of Pediatrics. 2009. Children's health topics: Secondhand tobacco smoke. www.aap.org/healthtopics/tobacco.cfm (accessed May 15, 2009).

Andrieu, N., D. F. Easton, J. Chang-Claude, M. A. Rookus, R. Brohet, E. Cardis, A. C. Antoniou, T. Wagner, J. Simard, G. Evans, S. Peock, J.-P. Fricker, C. Nogues, L. Van't Veer, F. E. van Leeuwen, and D. E. Goldgar. 2006. Effect of chest X-rays on the risk of breast cancer among BRCA1/2 mutation carriers in the International BRCA1/2 Carrier Cohort Study: A Report from the EMBRACE, GENEPSO, GEO-HEBON, and IBCCS Collaborators' Group. *Journal of Clinical Oncology* 24 (21):3361–66.

Antonuccio, D. O., W. G. Danton, G. Y. DeNelsky, R. P. Greenberg, and J. S. Gordon. 1999. Raising questions about antidepressants. *Psychotherapy and Psychosomatics* 68 (1):3–14.

Argyriou, A. A., E. Chroni, A. Koutras, J. Ellul, S. Papapetropoulos, G. Katsoulas, G. Iconomou, and H. P. Kalofonos. 2005. Vitamin E for prophylaxis against chemotherapy-induced neuropathy: A randomized controlled trial. *Neurology* 64 (1):26–31.

Armour, E. P., D. McEachern, Z. Wang, P. M. Corry, and A. Martinez. 1993. Sensitivity of human cells to mild hyperthermia. *Cancer Research* 53 (12):2740–44.

Arnetz, B. B., T. Akerstedt, L. Hillert, A. Lowden, N. Kuster, and C. Wiholm. 2007. The effects of 884 MHz GSM wireless communication signals on self-reported symptom and sleep (EEG): An experimental provocation study. Abstract. *Progress in Electromagnetic Research Symposium (PIERS)* 3 (7):1148–50, doi:10.2529/PIERS060907172142.

Aro, A., S. Männistö, I. Salminen, M. L. Ovaskainen, V. Kataja, and M. Uusitupa. 2000. Inverse association between dietary and serum conjugated linoleic acid and risk of breast cancer in postmenopausal women. *Nutrition and Cancer* 38 (2):151–57.

Arthur, J. R., R. C. McKenzie, and G. J. Beckett. 2003. Selenium in the immune system. *Journal of Nutrition* 133 (5 Suppl. 1):1457S–59.

Asfour, I. A., S. el Shazly, M. H. Fayek, H. M. Hegab, S. Raouf, and M. A. Moussa. 2006. Effect of high-dose sodium selenite therapy on polymorphonuclear leukocyte apoptosis in non-Hodgkin's lymphoma patients. *Biological Trace Element Research* 110 (1):19–32.

Augustin, L. S., J. Polesel, C. Bosetti, C. W. Kendall, C. La Vecchia, M. Parpinel, E. Conti, M. Montella, S. Franceschi, D. J. Jenkins, and L. Dal Maso. 2003. Dietary glycemic index, glycemic load, and ovarian cancer risk: A case-control study in Italy. *Annals of Oncology* 14 (1):78–84.

Avena, N. M., P. Rada, and B. G. Hoebel. 2008. Evidence for sugar addiction: Behavioral and neurochemical effects of intermittent, excessive sugar intake. *Neuroscience and Biobehavioral Reviews* 32 (1):20–39.

Babyak, M., J. A. Blumenthal, S. Herman, P. Khatri, M. Doraiswamy, K. Moore, W. E. Craighead, T. T. Baldewicz, and K. R. Krishnan. 2000. Exercise treatment for major depression: Maintenance of therapeutic benefit at 10 months. *Psychosomatic Medicine* 62 (5):633–38.

Bairati, I., F. Meyer, M. Gélinas, A. Fortin, A. Nabid, F. Brochet, J. P. Mercier, B. Têtu, F. Harel, B. Abdous, E. Vigneault, S. Vass, P. del Vecchio, and J. Roy. 2005. Randomized trial of antioxidant vitamins to prevent acute adverse effects of radiation therapy in head and neck cancer patients. *Journal of Clinical Oncology* 23 (24):5805–13.

Baker, B., S. L. Swezey, S. Guldan, D. Granatstein, and D. Chaney. 2005. *Organic Farming Compliance Handbook: A Resource Guide for Western Region Agricultural Professionals.* Davis, CA: University of California Agriculture and Natural Resources, Sustainable Agriculture Research and Education Program. www.sarep.ucdavis.edu/Organic/complianceguide/national.htm.

Barabás, J. and Z. Németh. 2006. The opinion of Hungarian Association of Oral and Maxillofacial Surgeons (*Magyar Arc-, Állcsont- és Szájsebészeti Társaság*) on the justification of supportive treatment of patients with tumorous diseases of the oral cavity. *Orvosi Hetilap (Hungarian Medical Journal)* 47(35): 1709-1711.

Bardia, A., L. C. Hartmann, C. M. Vachon, R. A. Vierkant, A. H. Wang, J. E. Olson, T. A. Sellers, and J. R. Cerhan. 2006. Recreational physical activity and risk of postmenopausal breast cancer based on hormone receptor status. *Archives of Internal Medicine* 166 (22):2478–83.

Barnard, R. J., J. H. Gonzales, M. E. Liva, and T. H. Ngo. 2006. Effects of a low-fat, high-fiber diet and exercise program on breast cancer risk factors in vivo and tumor cell growth and apoptosis in vitro. *Nutrition and Cancer* 55 (1):28–34.

Barton, D. L., G. S. Soori, B. Bauer, J. Sloan, P. A. Johnson, C. Figueras, S. Duane, S. Dakhil, H. Liu, and C. L. Loprinzi. 2007. A pilot, multi-dose, placebo-controlled evaluation of American ginseng (*Panax quinquefolius*) to improve cancer-related fatigue: NCCTG trial N03CA. *Journal of Clinical Oncology* 25 (18S):493s.

Battram, D. S., T. E. Graham, E. A. Richter, and F. Dela. 2005. The effect of caffeine on glucose kinetics in humans: Influence of adrenaline. *Journal of Physiology* 569 (Pt. 1):347–55.

Batty, D., and I. Thune. 2000. Does physical activity prevent cancer? Evidence suggests protection against colon cancer and probably breast cancer. *British Medical Journal* 321 (7274):1424–25.

Berger, W., M. V. Mendlowicz, C. Marques-Portella, G. Kinrys, L. F. Fontenelle, C. R. Marmar, and I. Figueira. 2009. Pharmacologic alternatives to antidepressants in posttraumatic stress disorder: A systematic review. *Progress in Neuro-Psychopharmacology and Biological Psychiatry* 33 (2):169–80.

Bergman, L., M. L. Beelen, M. P. Gallee, H. Hollema, J. Benraadt, and F. E. van Leeuwen. 2000. Risk and prognosis of endometrial cancer after tamoxifen for breast cancer: Comprehensive Cancer Centres' ALERT Group—Assessment of liver and endometrial cancer risk following tamoxifen. *Lancet* 356 (9233):881–87.

Bergström, A., P. Pisani, V. Tenet, A. Wolk, and H. O. Adami. 2001. Overweight as an avoidable cause of cancer in Europe. *International Journal of Cancer* 91 (3):421–30.

Bhattacharya, A., E. P. McCutcheon, E. Shvartz, and J. E. Greenleaf. 1980. Body acceleration distribution and O2 uptake in humans during running and jumping. *Journal of Applied Physiology* 49 (5):881–87.

Black, P. H. 2003. The inflammatory response is an integral part of the stress response: Implications for atherosclerosis, insulin resistance, type II diabetes, and metabolic syndrome X. *Brain, Behavior, and Immunity* 17 (5):350–64.

Block, G. 1991. Epidemiologic evidence regarding vitamin C and cancer. *American Journal of Clinical Nutrition* 54 (Suppl. 6):1310S–14.

Block, G., C. D. Jensen, E. P. Norkus, T. B. Dalvi, L. G. Wong, J. F. McManus, and M. L. Hudes. 2007. Usage patterns, health, and nutritional status of long-term multiple dietary supplement users: A cross-sectional study. *Nutrition Journal* 6:30.

Block, K. I., and M. N. Mead. 2003. Vitamin C in alternative cancer treatment: Historical background. *Integrative Cancer Therapies* 2 (2):147–54.

Bone, M. E., D. J. Wilkinson, J. R. Young, J. McNeil, and S. Charlton. 1990. Ginger root: A new antiemetic— The effect of ginger root on postoperative nausea and vomiting after major gynaecological surgery. *Anaesthesia* 45 (8):669–71.

Boros, L. G., M. Nichelatti, and Y. Shoenfeld. 2005. Fermented wheat germ extract (Avemar) in the treatment of cancer and autoimmune diseases. *Annals of the New York Academy of Sciences* 1051:529–42.

Boyle, P., and B. Levin. 2008. *World Cancer Report 2008*. Geneva, Switzerland: WHO (World Health Organization) Press.

Bremner, J. D., S. M. Southwick, D. R. Johnson, R. Yehuda, and D. S. Charney. 1993. Childhood physical abuse and combat-related posttraumatic stress disorder in Vietnam veterans. *American Journal of Psychiatry* 150 (2):235–39.

Bressler, B., L. F. Paszat, Z. Chen, D. M. Rothwell, C. Vinden, and L. Rabeneck. 2007. Rates of new or missed colorectal cancers after colonoscopy and their risk factors: A population-based analysis. *Gastroenterology* 132 (1):96–102.

Brickel, C. M. 1980. A review of the roles of pet animals in psychotherapy and with the elderly. *International Journal of Aging and Human Development* 12 (2):119–28.

Brizel, D. M., S. P. Scully, J. M. Harrelson, L. J. Layfield, J. M. Bean, L. R. Prosnitz, and M. W. Dewhirst. 1996. Tumor oxygenation predicts for the likelihood of distant metastases in human soft tissue sarcoma. *Cancer Research* 56 (5):941–43.

Brody, J. E. 1997. Puzzle in a Bottle: A Special Report—In vitamin mania, millions take a gamble on health. *New York Times*, October 26, U.S. section.

Brooks, J. D., E. J. Metter, D. W. Chan, L. J. Sokoll, P. Landis, W. G. Nelson, D. Muller, R. Andres, and H. B. Carter. 2001. Plasma selenium level before diagnosis and the risk of prostate cancer development. *Journal of Urology* 166 (6):2034–38.

Brooks, P. C., J. M. Lin, D. L. French, and J. P. Quigley. 1993. Subtractive immunization yields monoclonal antibodies that specifically inhibit metastasis. *Journal of Cell Biology* 122 (6):1351–59.

Brown, H. S., D. R. Bishop, and C. A. Rowan. 1984. The role of skin absorption as a route of exposure for volatile organic compounds (VOCs) in drinking water. *American Journal of Public Health* 74 (5):479–84.

Bull, J. M. 1982. Whole body hyperthermia as an anticancer agent. *CA: A Cancer Journal for Clinicians* 32 (2):123–28.

Bull, J. M., D. Lees, W. Schuette, J. Whang-Peng, R. Smith, G. Bynum, E. R. Atkinson, J. S. Gottdiener, H. R. Gralnick, T. H. Shawker, and V. T. DeVita, Jr. 1979. Whole body hyperthermia: A phase-I trial of a potential adjuvant to chemotherapy. *Annals of Internal Medicine* 90 (3):317–23.

Burton, G. W., M. G. Traber, R. V. Acuff, D. N. Walters, H. Kayden, L. Hughes, and K. U. Ingold. 1998. Human plasma and tissue alpha-tocopherol concentrations in response to supplementation with deuterated natural and synthetic vitamin E. *American Journal of Clinical Nutrition* 67 (4):669–84.

Calderon-Margalit, R., Y. Friedlander, R. Yanetz, K. Kleinhaus, M. C. Perrin, O. Manor, S. Harlap, and O. Paltiel. 2009. Cancer risk after exposure to treatments for ovulation induction. *American Journal of Epidemiology* 169 (3):365–75, doi:10.1093/aje/kwn318.

Cameron, E., and L. Pauling. 1976. Supplemental ascorbate in the supportive treatment of cancer: Prolongation of survival times in terminal human cancer. *Proceedings of the National Academy of Sciences* 73 (10):3685–89.

Cantor, K. P., C. F. Lynch, M. E. Hildesheim, M. Dosemeci, J. Lubin, M. Alavanja, and G. Craun. 1998. Drinking water source and chlorination byproducts: Risk of bladder cancer. *Epidemiology* 9 (1):21–28.

Cao, Y., and R. Cao. 1999. Angiogenesis inhibited by drinking tea. *Nature* 398 (6726):381.

Carlson, L. E., M. Speca, K. D. Patel, and E. Goodey. 2004. Mindfulness-based stress reduction in relation to quality of life, mood, symptoms of stress and levels of cortisol, dehydroepiandrosterone sulfate (DHEAS), and melatonin in breast and prostate cancer outpatients. *Psychoneuroendocrinology* 29 (4): 448–74.

Carpenter, D. O. 2005. Environmental contaminants and human health: The health effects of persistent toxic substances. *Fırat Tıp Dergisi* 10 (1):1–4.

Carroll, K. K., and H. T. Khor. 1975. Dietary fat in relation to tumorigenesis. *Progress in Biochemical Pharmacology* 10:308–53.

Cassileth, B. R., G. E. Deng, J. E. Gomez, P. A. Johnstone, N. Kumar, and A. J. Vickers; American College of Chest Physicians. 2007. Complementary therapies and integrative oncology in lung cancer: ACCP evidence-based clinical practice guidelines (2d ed.). *Chest* 132 (Suppl. 3):340S–54.

Cathcart, R. F. 1981. Vitamin C, titrating to bowel tolerance, anascorbemia, and acute induced scurvy. *Medical Hypotheses* 7 (11):1359–76.

Cavalieri, E. L., D. E. Stack, P. D. Devanesan, R. Todorovic, I. Dwivedy, S. Higginbotham, S. L. Johansson, K. D. Patil, M. L. Gross, J. K. Gooden, R. Ramanathan, R. L. Cerny, and E. G. Rogan. 1997. Molecular origin of cancer: Catechol estrogen-3,4-quinones as endogenous tumor initiators. *Proceedings of the National Academy of Sciences* 94 (20):10937–942.

Centers for Disease Control and Prevention (CDC). 2005. *National Report on Human Exposure to Environmental Chemicals*. 3rd report. Atlanta, GA: Department of Health and Human Services, CDC. www.cdc.gov/exposurereport/.

Chakravarty, A. K., and H. Yasmin. 2005. Alcoholic turmeric extract simultaneously activating murine lymphocytes and inducing apoptosis of Ehlrich ascitic carcinoma cells. *International Immunopharmacology* 5 (10):1574–81.

Chami, N., S. Bennis, F. Chami, A. Aboussekhra, and A. Remmal. 2005. Study of anticandidal activity of carvacrol and eugenol in vitro and in vivo. *Oral Microbiology and Immunology* 20 (2):106–11.

Chan, J. M., C. N. Holick, M. F. Leitzmann, E. B. Rimm, W. C. Willett, M. J. Stampfer, and E. L. Giovannucci. 2006. Diet after diagnosis and the risk of prostate cancer progression, recurrence, and death (United States). *Cancer Causes and Control* 17 (2):199–208.

Chan, J. M., M. J. Stampfer, E. Giovannucci, P. H. Gann, J. Ma, P. Wilkinson, C. H. Hennekens, and M. Pollak. 1998. Plasma insulin-like growth factor-1 and prostate cancer risk: A prospective study. *Science* 279 (5350):563–66.

Chavarro, J., M. Stampfer, H. Campos, T. Kurth, W. Willett, and J. Ma. 2006. A prospective study of blood trans-fatty acid levels and risk of prostate cancer. *Proceedings of the American Association for Cancer Research* 47 (1):943.

Chen, K., and R. Yeung. 2002. A Review of qigong therapy for cancer treatment. *Journal of International Society of Life Information Science (ISLIS)* 20 (2):532–42.

Chen, Q., M. G. Espey, A. Y. Sun, C. Pooput, K. L. Kirk, M. C. Krishna, D. B. Khosh, J. Drisko, and M. Levine. 2008. Pharmacologic doses of ascorbate act as a prooxidant and decrease growth of aggressive tumor xenografts in mice. *Proceedings of the National Academy of Sciences* 105 (32):11105–09.

Cheney, G. 1949. Rapid healing of peptic ulcers in patients receiving fresh cabbage juice. *California Medicine* 70 (1):10–15.

Chinery, R., J. A. Brockman, M. O. Peeler, Y. Shyr, R. D. Beauchamp, and R. J. Coffey. 1997. Antioxidants enhance the cytotoxicity of chemotherapeutic agents in colorectal cancer: A p53-independent induction of p21WAF1/CIP1 via C/EBPbeta. *Nature Medicine* 3 (11):1233–41.

Chinn, D. O. 2005. Transrectal HIFU: The Next Generation? *Prostate Cancer Research Institute Insights* 8 (1):14.

Chlebowski, R. T., L. Bulcavage, M. Grosvenor, E. Oktay, J. B. Block, J. S. Chlebowski, I. Ali, and R. Elashoff. 1990. Hydrazine sulfate influence on nutritional status and survival in non-small-cell lung cancer. *Journal of Clinical Oncology* 8 (1):9–15.

Cho, R. W., X. Wang, M. Diehn, K. Shedden, G. Y. Chen, G. Sherlock, A. Gurney, J. Lewicki, and M. F. Clarke. 2008. Isolation and molecular characterization of cancer stem cells in MMTV-Wnt-1 murine breast tumors. *Stem Cells* 26 (2):364 –71.

Christensen, A. J., D. L. Edwards, J. S. Wiebe, E. G. Benotsch, L. McKelvey, M. Andrews, and D. M. Lubaroff. 1996. Effect of verbal self-disclosure on natural killer cell activity: Moderating influence of cynical hostility. *Psychosomatic Medicine* 58 (2):150–55.

Clark, L. C., G. F. Combs Jr., B. W. Turnbull, E. H. Slate, D. K. Chalker, J. Chow, L. S. Davis, R. A. Glover, G. F. Graham, E. G. Gross, A. Krongrad, J. L. Lesher Jr., H. K. Park, B. B. Sanders Jr., C. L. Smith, and J. R. Taylor; Nutritional Prevention of Cancer Study Group. 1996. Effects of selenium supplementation for cancer prevention in patients with carcinoma of the skin: A randomized controlled trial. *Journal of the American Medical Association* 276 (24):1957–63.

Clark, M. M., J. M. Bostwick, and T. A. Rummans. 2003. Group and individual treatment strategies for distress in cancer patients. *Mayo Clinic Proceedings* 78 (12):1538–43.

Clement-Jones, V., L. McLoughlin, S. Tomlin, G. M. Besser, L. H. Rees, and H. L. Wen. 1980. Increased beta-endorphin but not met-enkephalin levels in human cerebrospinal fluid after acupuncture for recurrent pain. *Lancet* 2 (8201):946–49.

Cohen, L. A., C. Aliaga, B. Pittman, and E. L. Wynder. 1999. Oral enzyme therapy and experimental rat mammary tumor metastasis. *Life Sciences* 65 (24):2603–14.

Cole, W. H. 1981. Efforts to explain spontaneous regression of cancer. *Journal of Surgical Oncology* 17 (3):201–09.

Combs, A. B., J. Y. Choe, D. H. Truong, and K. Folkers. 1977. Reduction by coenzyme $Q_{10}$ of the acute toxicity of adriamycin in mice. *Research Communications in Chemical Pathology and Pharmacology* 18 (3):565–68.

Cordain, L., S. B. Eaton, A. Sebastian, N. Mann, S. Lindeberg, B. A. Watkins, J. H. O'Keefe, J. Brand-Miller. 2005. Origins and evolution of the Western diet: Health implications for the 21st century. *American Journal of Clinical Nutrition* 81 (2):341–54.

Costanzo, E. S., S. K. Lutgendorf, A. K. Sood, B. Anderson, J. Sorosky, and D. M. Lubaroff. 2005. Psychosocial factors and interleukin-6 among women with advanced ovarian cancer. *Cancer* 104 (2):305–13.

Cotterchio, M. N. Kreiger, G. Darlington, and A. Steingart. 2000. Antidepressant medication use and breast cancer risk. *American Journal of Epidemiology* 151 (10):951–57.

Cottreau, C. M., R. B. Ness, and A. M. Kriska. 2000. Physical activity and reduced risk of ovarian cancer. *Obstetrics and Gynecology* 96 (4):609–14.

Cottreau, C. M., R. B. Ness, F. Modugno, G. O. Allen, and M. T. Goodman. 2003. Endometriosis and its treatment with danazol or lupron in relation to ovarian cancer. *Clinical Cancer Research* 9 (14):5142–44.

Cowawintaweewat, S., S. Manoromana, H. Sriplung, T. Khuhaprema, P. Tongtawe, P. Tapchaisri, and W. Chaicumpa. 2006. Prognostic improvement of patients with advanced liver cancer after active hexose correlated compound (AHCC) treatment. *Asian Pacific Journal of Allergy and Immunology* 24 (1):34–45.

Cox, A. J., D. B. Pyne, P. U. Saunders, and P. A. Fricker. 2008. Oral administration of the probiotic Lactobacillus fermentum VRI-003 and mucosal immunity in endurance athletes. *British Journal of Sports Medicine*, February 13, doi:10.1136/bjsm.2007.044628.

Creagan, E. T., C. G. Moertel, J. R. O'Fallon, A. J. Schutt, M. J. O'Connell, J. Rubin, and S. Frytak. 1979. Failure of high-dose vitamin C (ascorbic acid) therapy to benefit patients with advanced cancer: A controlled trial. *New England Journal of Medicine* 301 (13):687–90.

Creech, Jr., J. L., and M. N. Johnson. 1974. Angiosarcoma of liver in the manufacture of polyvinyl chloride. *Journal of Occupational Medicine* 16 (3):150–51.

Cui, H., M. Cruz-Correa, F. M. Giardiello, D. F. Hutcheon, D. R. Kafonek, S. Brandenburg, Y. Wu, X. He, N. R. Powe, and A. P. Feinberg. 2003a. Loss of IGF2 imprinting: A potential marker of colorectal cancer risk. *Science* 299 (5613):1753–55.

Cui, Z., M. C. Willingham, A. M. Hicks, M. A. Alexander-Miller, T. D. Howard, G. A. Hawkins, M. S. Miller, H. M. Weir, W. Du, and C. J. DeLong. 2003b. Spontaneous regression of advanced cancer: Identification of a unique genetically determined, age-dependent trait in mice. *Proceedings of the National Academy of Sciences* 100 (11):6682–87.

Curtis, R. E., D. M. Freedman, E. Ron, L. A. G. Ries, D. G. Hacker, B. K. Edwards, M. A. Tucker, and J. F. Fraumeni, Jr., eds. 2006. New malignancies among cancer survivors: SEER cancer registries, 1973–2000. National Cancer Institute, *NIH Publ. No. 05-5302.* Bethesda, MD.

Dale, P. S., C. P. Tamhanker, D. George, and G. V. Daftary. 2001. Co-medication with hydrolytic enzymes in radiation therapy of uterine cervix: Evidence of the reduction of acute side effects. *Cancer Chemotherapy and Pharmacology* 47 Suppl.:S29–34.

Damasio, A. R., T. J. Grabowski, A. Bechara, H. Damasio, L. L. Ponto, J. Parvizi, and R. D. Hichwa. 2000. Subcortical and cortical brain activity during the feeling of self-generated emotions. *Nature Neuroscience* 3 (10):1049–56.

Davidson, P. R., and K. C. Parker. 2001. Eye Movement Desensitization and Reprocessing (EMDR): A meta-analysis. *Journal of Consulting and Clinical Psychology* 69 (2):305–16.

Davis, D. L., and B. H. Magee. 1979. Cancer and industrial chemical production. *Science* 206 (4425):1356–58.

Davis, J. N., N. Muqim, M. Bhuiyan, O. Kucuk, K. J. Pienta, and F. H. Sarkar. 2000. Inhibition of prostate specific antigen expression by genistein in prostate cancer cells. *International Journal of Oncology.* 16 (6):1091–97.

Davis, L., and G. Kuttan. 1998. Suppressive effect of cyclophosphamide-induced toxicity by *Withania somnifera* extract in mice. *Journal of Ethnopharmacology* 62 (3):209–14.

Dekker, J. M., E. G. Schouten, P. Klootwijk, J. Pool, C. A. Swenne, and D. Kromhout. 1997. Heart rate variability from short electrocardiographic recordings predicts mortality from all causes in middle-aged and elderly men: The Zutphen Study. *American Journal of Epidemiology* 145 (10):899–908.

Demark-Wahnefried, W., D. T. Price, T. J. Polascik, C. N. Robertson, E. E. Anderson, D. F. Paulson, P. J. Walther, M. Gannon, and R. T. Vollmer. 2001. Pilot study of dietary fat restriction and flaxseed supplementation in men with prostate cancer before surgery: Exploring the effects on hormonal levels, prostate-specific antigen, and histopathologic features. *Urology* 58 (1):47–52.

Demicheli, R., M. W. Retsky, W. J. Hrushesky, M. Baum, and I. D. Gukas. 2008. The effects of surgery on tumor growth: A century of investigations. *Annals of Oncology* 19 (11):1821–28.

Demidov, L. V., L. V. Manzjuk, G. Y. Kharkevitch, E. V. Artamonova, and N. A. Pirogova. 2002. The antimetastatic effect of Avemar in high-risk melanoma patients. 18th UICC International Cancer Congress, Oslo, Norway, June 30–July 5. Abstract. *International Journal of Cancer* 100 (S13):408.

Dunn, S. E., R. A. Hardman, F. W. Kari, and J. C. Barrett. 1997. Insulin-like growth factor 1 (IGF-1) alters drug sensitivity of HBL 100 human breast cancer cells by inhibition of apoptosis induced by diverse anticancer drugs. *Cancer Research* 57 (13):2687–93.

Duraffourd, C., and J. C. Lapraz. 2002. *Traité de phytothérapie clinique: Endobiogénie et médecine (Treatise on Clinical Phytotherapy: Endobiogeny and Medicine)*. Paris: Editions Masson.

Durlach, J., M. Bara, A. Guiet-Bara, and P. Collery. 1986. Relationship between magnesium, cancer, and carcinogenic or anticancer metals. *Anticancer Research* 6 (6):1353–61.

Dvorak, H. F. 1986. Tumors: Wounds that do not heal—Similarities between tumor stroma generation and healing. *New England Journal of Medicine* 315 (26):1650–59.

Ehret, C. F., J. C. Meinert, K. R. Groh, K. W. Dobra, and G. A. Antipa. 1999. Circadian regulation: Growth kinetics of the infradian cell. In *Growth kinetics and biochemical regulation of normal and malignant cells: A collection of papers presented at the twenty-ninth annual Symposium on Fundamental Cancer Research, 1976*, ed. B. Drewinko and R. M. Humphrey. Baltimore: Williams and Wilkins 49–76.

Eliaz, I., A. T. Hotchkiss, M. L. Fishman, and D. Rode. 2006. The effect of modified citrus pectin on urinary excretion of toxic elements. *Phytotherapy Research* 20 (10):859–64.

Elmore, J. G., M. B. Barton, V. M. Moceri, S. Polk, P. J. Arena, and S. W. Fletcher. 1998. Ten-year risk of false positive screening mammograms and clinical breast examinations. *New England Journal of Medicine* 338 (16):1089–96.

Endres, S., R. Ghorbani, V. E. Kelley, K. Georgilis, G. Lonnemann, J. W. van der Meer, J. G. Cannon, T. S. Rogers, M. S. Klempner, P. C. Weber, E. J. Schaefer, S. M. Wolff, and C. A. Dinarello. 1989. The effect of dietary supplementation with n-3 polyunsaturated fatty acids on the synthesis of interleukin-1 and tumor necrosis factor by mononuclear cells. New England Journal of Medicine 320 (5):265–71.

Environmental Working Group (EWG). 2005. Body burden: The pollution in newborns. Washington, DC. http://archive.ewg.org/reports/bodyburden2/execsumm.php (accessed May 16, 2009).

European Food Safety Authority. 2008. Opinion on mixed tocopherols, tocotrienol tocopherol, and tocotrienols as sources for vitamin E added as a nutritional substance in food supplements: Scientific opinion of the Panel on Food Additives, Flavourings, Processing aids, and Materials in Contact with Food (AFC). *European Food Safety Authority Journal* 640:1–34.

Evangelou, A., G. Kalpouzos, S. Karkabounas, R. Liasko, A. Nonni, D. Stefanou, and G. Kallistratos. 1997. Dose-related preventive and therapeutic effects of antioxidants-anticarcinogens on experimentally induced malignant tumors in Wistar rats. *Cancer Letters* 115 (1):105–11.

Federico, A., P. Iodice, P. Federico, A. del Rio, M. C. Mellone, G. Catalano, and P. Federico. 2001. Effects of selenium and zinc supplementation on nutritional status in patients with cancer of digestive tract. *European Journal of Clinical Nutrition* 55 (4):293–97.

Fernandez, M. F., C. Aguilar-Garduño, J. M. Molina-Molina, J. P. Arrebola, and N. Olea. 2008. The total effective xenoestrogen burden, a biomarker of exposure to xenoestrogen mixtures, is predicted by the (anti)estrogenicity of its components. *Reproductive Toxicology* 26 (1):8–12.

Fernstrom, J. D., R. J. Wurtman, B. Hammarstrom-Wiklund, W. M. Rand, H. N. Munro, and C. S. Davidson. 1979. Diurnal variations in plasma concentrations of tryptophan, tyrosine, and other neutral amino acids: Effect of dietary protein intake. *American Journal of Clinical Nutrition* 32 (9):1912–22.

Ferrández, M. D., R. Correa, M. del Rio, and M. de la Fuente. 1999. Effects in vitro of several antioxidants on the natural killer function of aging mice. *Experimental Gerontology* 34 (5):675–85.

Ferreira, P. R., J. F. Fleck, A. Diehl, D. Barletta, A. Braga-Filho, A. Barletta, and L. Ilha. 2004. Protective effect of alpha-tocopherol in head and neck cancer radiation-induced mucositis: A double-blind randomized trial. *Head and Neck* 26 (4):313–21.

Ferrell, V. 1998. *Alternative Cancer Remedies: Facts for Historians and Medical Researchers.* Beersheba Springs, TN: Pilgrims Books.

Fiers, W., R. Beyaert, W. Declercq, and P. Vandenabeele. 1999. More than one way to die: Apoptosis, necrosis, and reactive oxygen damage. *Oncogene* 18 (54):7719–30.

Filov, V. A., M. L. Gershanovich, L. A. Danova, and B. A. Ivin. 1995. Experience of the treatment with Sehydrin (Hydrazine Sulfate, HS) in the advanced cancer patients. *Investigational New Drugs* 13 (1):89–97.

Folkers, K., R. Brown, W. V. Judy, and M. Morita. 1993. Survival of cancer patients on therapy with coenzyme Q10. *Biochemical and Biophysical Research Communications* 192 (1):241–45.

Folkman, J., E. Merler, C. Abernathy, and G. Williams. 1971. Isolation of a tumor factor responsible for angiogenesis. *Journal of Experimental Medicine* 133 (2):275–88.

Fonorow, O. 2007. The nature of vitamin C: The position of the Vitamin C Foundation on natural vitamin C and so-called vitamin C-complex. *Townsend Letter* 293:90–97.

Fontana, L., S. Klein, and J. O. Holloszy. 2006. Long-term low-protein, low-calorie diet and endurance exercise modulate metabolic factors associated with cancer risk. *American Journal of Clinical Nutrition* 84 (6):1456–62.

Ford, E. S. 2002. Does exercise reduce inflammation? Physical activity and C-reactive protein among U.S. adults. *Epidemiology* 13 (5):561–68.

Foster-Powell, K., S. H. Holt, and J. C. Brand-Miller. 2002. International table of glycemic index and glycemic load values: 2002. *American Journal of Clinical Nutrition* 76 (1):5–56.

Fournié, G. J., A. Saoudi, P. Druet, and L. Pelletier. 2002. Th2-type immunopathological manifestations induced by mercury chloride or gold salts in the rat: Signal transduction pathways, cellular mechanisms, and genetic control. *Autoimmunity Reviews* 1 (4):205–12.

Franceschi, S., L. dal Maso, L. Augustin, E. Negri, M. Parpinel, P. Boyle, D. J. Jenkins, and C. la Vecchia. 2001. Dietary glycemic load and colorectal cancer risk. *Annals of Oncology* 12 (2):1173–78.

Friedenreich, C. M., and M. R. Orenstein. 2002. Physical activity and cancer prevention: Etiologic evidence and biological mechanisms. *Journal of Nutrition* 132 (11 Suppl.):3456S–64.

Frisch, R. E., G. Wyshak, N. L. Albright, T. E. Albright, I. Schiff, K. P. Jones, J. Witschi, E. Shiang, E. Koff, and M. Marguglio. 1985. Lower prevalence of breast cancer and cancers of the reproductive system among former college athletes compared to non-athletes. *British Journal of Cancer* 52 (6):885–91.

Frisina, P. G., J. C. Borod, and S. J. Lepore. 2004. A meta-analysis of the effects of written emotional disclosure on the health outcomes of clinical populations. *Journal of Nervous and Mental Disease* 192 (9):629–34.

Funahashi, H., T. Imai, Y. Tanaka, J. Tobinaga, M. Wada, T. Morita, F. Yamada, K. Tsukamura, M. Oiwa, T. Kikumori, T. Narita, and H. Takagi. 1996. Suppressive effect of iodine on DMBA-induced breast tumor growth in the rat. *Journal of Surgical Oncology* 61 (3):209–13.

Gamet-Payrastre, L., P. Li, S. Lumeau, G. Cassar, M. A. Dupont, S. Chevolleau, N. Gasc, J. Tulliez, and F. Tercé. 2000. Sulforaphane, a naturally occurring isothiocyanate, induces cell cycle arrest and apoptosis in HT29 human colon cancer cells. *Cancer Research* 60 (5):1426–33.

Gao, X., D. Deeb, H. Jiang, Y. B. Liu, S. A. Dulchavsky, and S. C. Gautam. 2005. Curcumin differentially sensitizes malignant glioma cells to TRAIL/Apo2L-mediated apoptosis through activation of procaspases and release of cytochrome c from mitochondria. *Journal of Experimental Therapeutics and Oncology* 5 (1):39–48.

Gao, Y., D. Zhang, B. Sun, H. Fujii, K. Kosuna, and Z. Yin. 2006. Active hexose correlated compound enhances tumor surveillance through regulating both innate and adaptive immune responses. *Cancer Immunology, Immunotherapy* 55 (10):1258–66.

Garami, M., D. Schuler, M. Babosa, G. Borgulya, P. Hauser, J. Müller, A. Paksy, E. Szabó, M. Hidvégi, and G. Fekete. 2004. Fermented wheat germ extract reduces chemotherapy-induced febrile neutropenia in pediatric cancer patients. *Journal of Pediatric Hematology/Oncology* 26 (10):631–35.

Garcia-Alejo Hernández, R., M. J. Martín de Miguel, J. M. Seoane Lestón, M. A. Romero Méndez, and G. C. Esparza Gómez. 1989. Radioprotective effect of ascorbic acid on oral structures in patients with cancer of the head and neck. [In Spanish.] *Avances en odontoestomatologia* 5 (7):469–72.

Gardner, S. F., M. A. Marx, L. M. White, M. C. Granberry, D. R. Skelton, and V. A. Fonseca. 1997. Combination of low-dose niacin and pravastatin improves the lipid profile in diabetic patients without compromising glycemic control. *Annals of Pharmacotherapy* 31 (6):677–82.

Garland, C. F., E. D. Gorham, S. B. Mohr, W. B. Grant, E. L. Giovannucci, M. Lipkin, H. Newmark, M. F. Holick, and F. C. Garland. 2007. Vitamin D and prevention of breast cancer: Pooled analysis. *Journal of Steroid Biochemistry and Molecular Biology* 103 (3–5):708–11.

Garton, G. A. 1960. Fatty acid composition of the lipids of pasture grasses. *Nature* 187:511–12.

Gershon, M. D. 1998. *The Second Brain: The Scientific Basis of Gut Instinct and a Groundbreaking New Understanding of Nervous Disorders of the Stomach and Intestines.* New York: HarperCollins.

Ghoneum, M., M. Wimbley, F. Salem, A. McKlain, N. Attalah, and G. Gill. 1995. Immunomodulatory and anticancer effects of Active Hemicellulose Compound (AHCC). *International Journal of Immunotherapy* X1 (1):23–28.

Giovannucci, E., M. Leitzmann, D. Spiegelman, E. B. Rimm, G. A. Colditz, M. J. Stampfer, and W. C. Willett. 1998a. A prospective study of physical activity and prostate cancer in male health professionals. *Cancer Research* 58 (22):5117–22.

Giovannucci, E., M. J. Stampfer, G. A. Colditz, D. J. Hunter, C. Fuchs, B. A. Rosner, F. E. Speizer, and W. C. Willett. 1998b. Multivitamin use, folate, and colon cancer in women in the Nurses' Health Study. *Annals of Internal Medicine* 129 (7):517–24.

Goodin, M. G., and R. J. Rosengren. 2003. Epigallocatechin gallate modulates CYP450 isoforms in the female Swiss-Webster mouse. *Toxicological Sciences* 76 (2):262–70.

Goodwin, P. J., M. Ennis, K. I. Pritchard, J. Koo, and N. Hood. 2008. Frequency of vitamin D (Vit D) deficiency at breast cancer (BC) diagnosis and association with risk of distant recurrence and death in a prospective cohort study of T1-3, NO-1, MO B. Abstract. *Journal of Clinical Oncology* 26 (15S [May 20 Suppl.]):511.

Gorham, E. D., C. F. Garland, F. C. Garland, W. B. Grant, S. B. Mohr, M. Lipkin, H. L. Newmark, E. Giovannucci, M. Wei, and M. F. Holick. 2007. Optimal vitamin D status for colorectal cancer prevention: A quantitative meta analysis. *American Journal of Preventive Medicine* 32 (3):210–16.

Gosline, A. 2006. Health: Why fast foods are bad, even in moderation. *NewScientist*. www.newscientist.com/article/dn9318-why-fast-foods-are-bad-even-in-moderation.html.

Gottlieb, N. 1999. Cancer treatment and vitamin C: The debate lingers. *Journal of the National Cancer Institute* 91 (24):2073–75.

Goud, V. K., K. Polasa, and K. Krishnaswamy. 1993. Effect of turmeric on xenobiotic metabolising enzymes. *Plant Foods for Human Nutrition* 44 (1):87–92.

Gould, J. M. 1986. *Quality of Life in American Neighborhoods: Levels of Affluence, Toxic Waste, and Cancer Mortality in Residential Zip Code Areas*. Boulder, CO: Westview Press.

Grant, W. B. 2004. The role of ultraviolet-B (UVB) radiation (290–315 nm) and vitamin D in reducing the risk of cancer. Sunlight, Nutrition, and Health Research Center (SUNARC), www.sunarc.org/papers.htm#cancer (accessed May 14, 2009).

Grant, W. B., and M. F. Holick. 2005. Benefits and requirements of vitamin D for optimal health: A review. *Alternative Medicine Review* 10 (2):94–111.

Grazzi, L., F. Andrasik, S. Usai, and G. Bussone. 2005. Magnesium as a treatment for paediatric tension-type headache: A clinical replication series. *Neurological Sciences* 25 (6):338–41.

Grevelman, E. G., and W. P. M. Breed. 2005. Prevention of chemotherapy-induced hair loss by scalp cooling. *Annals of Oncology* 16 (3):352–58.

Groopman, J. 1998. Annals of medicine: Dr. Fair's tumor. *New Yorker*, October 26.

Grossman, P., L. Niemann, S. Schmidt, and H. Walach. 2004. Mindfulness-based stress reduction and health benefits: A meta-analysis. *Journal of Psychosomatic Research* 57 (1):35–43.

Gu, J. W., G. Gadonski, J. Wang, I. Makey, and T. H. Adair. 2004. Exercise increases endostatin in circulation of healthy volunteers. *BMC Physiology* 4:2.

Guadagnino, E., L. Gramiccioni, M. Denaro, and M. Baldini. 1998. Co-operative study on the release of lead from crystalware. *Packaging Technology and Science* 11 (2):45–57.

Gupta, S., and J. Prakash. 2009. Studies on Indian green leafy vegetables for their antioxidant activity. *Plant Foods for Human Nutrition* 64 (1):39–45.

Hager, K., A. Marahrens, M. Kenklies, P. Riederer, and G. Münch. 2001. Alpha-lipoic acid as a new treatment option for Alzheimer type dementia. *Archives of Gerontology and Geriatrics* 32 (3):275–82.

Handelman, G. J., W. L. Epstein, J. Peerson, D. Spiegelman, L. J. Machlin, and E. A. Dratz. 1994. Human adipose alpha-tocopherol and gamma-tocopherol kinetics during and after 1 y of alpha-tocopherol supplementation. *American Journal of Clinical Nutrition* 59 (5):1025–32.

Hannes, B., H. B. Stähelin, K. F. Gey, M. Eichholzer, E. Lüdin, F. Bernasconi, J. Thumeysen, and G. Brubacher. 1991. Plasma antioxidant vitamins and subsequent cancer mortality in the 12-year follow-up of the prospective Basel Study. *American Journal of Epidemiology* 133 (8):766–75.

Hansen, C. J., L. C. Stevens, and J. R. Coast. 2001. Exercise duration and mood state: How much is enough to feel better? *Health Psychology* 20 (4):267–75.

Hara, M., T. Hanaoka, M. Kobayashi, T. Otani, H. Y. Adachi, A. Montani, S. Natsukawa, K. Shaura, Y. Koizumi, Y. Kasuga, T. Matsuzawa, T. Ikekawa, S. Sasaki, and S. Tsugane. 2003. Cruciferous vegetables, mushrooms, and gastrointestinal cancer risks in a multicenter, hospital-based case-control study in Japan. *Nutrition and Cancer* 46 (2):138–47.

Hasegawa, Y., N. Kubota, T. Inagaki, and N. Shinagawa. 2001. Music therapy-induced alternations in natural killer cell count and function. [In Japanese.] *Japanese Journal of Geriatrics* 38 (2):201–04.

Heim, C., D. J. Newport, S. Heit, Y. P. Graham, M. Wilcox, R. Bonsall, A. H. Miller, and C. B. Nemeroff. 2000. Pituitary-adrenal and autonomic responses to stress in women after sexual and physical abuse in childhood. *Journal of the American Medical Association* 284 (5):592–97.

Heini, A. F., and R. L. Weinsier. 1997. Divergent trends in obesity and fat intake patterns: The American paradox. *American Journal of Medicine* 102 (3):259–64.

Helzlsouer, K. J., H. Y. Huang, A. J. Alberg, S. Hoffman, A. Burke, E. P. Norkus, J. S. Morris, and G. W. Comstock. 2000. Association between alpha-tocopherol, gamma-tocopherol, selenium, and subsequent prostate cancer. *Journal of the National Cancer Institute* 92 (24):2018–23.

Hernandez-Reif, M., T. Field, G. Ironson, J. Beutler, Y. Vera, J. Hurley, M. A. Fletcher, S. Schanberg, C. Kuhn, and M. Fraser. 2005. Natural killer cells and lymphocytes increase in women with breast cancer following massage therapy. *International Journal of Neuroscience* 115 (4):495–510.

Hirose, A., E. Sato, H. Fujii, B. Sun, H. Nishioka, O.I. Aruoma. 2007. The influence of active hexose correlated compound (AHCC) on cisplatin-evoked chemotherapeutic and side effects in tumor-bearing mice. *Toxicology and Applied Pharmacology* 222(2):152-158.

Höckel, M., C. Knoop, K. Schlenger, B. Vorndran, E. Baussmann, M. Mitze, P. G. Knapstein, and P. Vaupel. 1993. Intratumoral pO2 predicts survival in advanced cancer of the uterine cervix. *Radiotherapy and Oncology* 26 (1):45–50.

Hogan, P. G., and A. Basten. 1988. What are killer cells and what do they do? *Blood Reviews* 2 (1):50–58.

Holmes, M. D., W. Y. Chen, D. Feskanich, C. H. Kroenke, and G. A. Colditz. 2005. Physical activity and survival after breast cancer diagnosis. *Journal of the American Medical Association* 293 (20):2479–86.

Hooning, M. J., A. Botma, B. M. Aleman, M. H. Baaijens, H. Bartelink, J. G. Klijn, C. W. Taylor, and F. E. van Leeuwen. 2007. Long-term risk of cardiovascular disease in 10-year survivors of breast cancer. *Journal of the National Cancer Institute* 99 (5):365–75.

Horvath, G., G. af Klinteberg Järverud, S. Järverud, and I. Horváth. 2008. Human ovarian carcinomas detected by specific odor. *Integrative Cancer Therapies* 7 (2):76–80.

Hosoe, K., M. Kitano, H. Kishida, H. Kubo, K. Fujii, and M. Kitahara. 2007. Study on safety and bioavailability of ubiquinol (Kaneka QH) after single and 4-week multiple oral administration to healthy volunteers. *Regulatory Toxicology and Pharmacology* 47 (1):19–28.

Hsing, A. W., A. P. Chokkalingam, Y. T. Gao, M. P. Madigan, J. Deng, G. Gridley, and J. F. Fraumeni, Jr. 2002. Allium vegetables and risk of prostate cancer: A population-based study. *Journal of the National Cancer Institute* 94 (21):1648–51.

Human Genome Project Information. 2008. Oak Ridge National Laboratory, Oak Ridge, TN, www.ornl.gov/sci/techresources/Human_Genome/medicine/assist.shtml (accessed May 11, 2009).

Iarussi, D., U. Auricchio, A. Agretto, A. Murano, M. Giuliano, F. Casale, P. Indolfi, and A. Iacono. 1994. Protective effect of coenzyme Q10 on anthracyclines cardiotoxicity: Control study in children with acute lymphoblastic leukemia and non-Hodgkin lymphoma. *Molecular Aspects of Medicine* 15 (Supplement): S207–12.

Illman, J., R. Corringham, D. Robinson Jr., H. M. Davis, J. F. Rossi, D. Cella, and M. Trikha. 2005. Are inflammatory cytokines the common link between cancer-associated cachexia and depression? *Journal of Supportive Oncology* 3 (1):37–50.

Ingram, D. 1994. Diet and subsequent survival in women with breast cancer. *British Journal of Cancer* 69 (3):592–95.

Innis, S. M. 2007. Dietary (n-3) fatty acids and brain development. *Journal of Nutrition* 137 (4):855–59.

Inoue, S., and M. Kabaya. 1989. Biological activities caused by far-infrared radiation. *International Journal of Biometeorology* 33 (3):145–50.

Inoue-Sakurai, C., S. Maruyama, and K. Morimoto. 2000. Posttraumatic stress and lifestyles are associated with natural killer cell activity in victims of the Hanshin-Awaji earthquake in Japan. *Preventive Medicine* 31 (5):467–73.

Institute of Medicine. 2002. *Dietary Reference Intakes for Vitamin A, Vitamin K, Arsenic, Boron, Chromium, Copper, Iodine, Iron, Manganese, Molybdenum, Nickel, Silicon, Vanadium, and Zinc.* Washington, DC: National Academies Press.

International AHCC Research Association. 2006. Proceedings of the International AHCC Research Symposium, Sapporo, Japan.

International Programme on Chemical Safety. 1991. *Health and Safety Guide No. 62: Nickel, Nickel Carbonyl, and some Nickel Compounds Health and Safety Guide.* Geneva: World Health Organization. www.inchem.org/documents/hsg/hsg/hsg062.htm#SectionNumber:2.3.

Ip, C., J. A. Scimeca, and H. J. Thompson. 1994. Conjugated linoleic acid: A powerful anticarcinogen from animal fat sources. *Cancer* 74 (3 Suppl.):1050–54.

Ironson, G., T. Field, F. Scafidi, M. Hashimoto, M. Kumar, A. Kumar, A. Price, A. Goncalves, I. Burman, C. Tetenman, R. Patarca, and M. A. Fletcher. 1986. Massage therapy is associated with enhancement of the immune system's cytotoxic capacity. *International Journal of Neuroscience* 84 (1–4):205–17.

Ironson, G., C. Wynings, N. Schneiderman, A. Baum, M. Rodriguez, D. Greenwood, C. Benight, M. Antoni, A. LaPerriere, H. S. Huang, N. Klimas, and M. A. Fletcher. 1997. Posttraumatic stress symptoms, intrusive thoughts, loss, and immune function after Hurricane Andrew. *Psychosomatic Medicine* 59 (2):128–41.

Ito, C., K. Yamaguchi, Y. Shibutani, K. Suzuki, Y. Yamazaki, H. Komachi, H. Ohnishi, and H. Fujimura. 1979. Anti-inflammatory actions of proteases, bromelain, trypsin, and their mixed preparations. [In Japanese.] *Folia Pharmacologica Japonica* 75 (3):227.

Jakab, F., Y. Shoenfeld, A. Balogh, M. Nichelatti, A. Hoffmann, Z. Kahán, K. Lapis, A. Mayer, P. Sápy, F. Szentpépery, A. Telekes, L. Thurzó, A. Vágvölgyi, and M. Hidvégi. 2003. A medical nutriment has supportive value in the treatment of colorectal cancer. *British Journal of Cancer* 89 (3):465–69.

Jemal, A., R. Siegel, E. Ward, T. Murray, J. Xu, C. Smigal, and M. J. Thun. 2006. Cancer Statistics 2006. *CA: A Cancer Journal for Clinicians* 56 (2):106–30.

John, E. M., G. G. Schwartz, J. Koo, D. van den Berg, and S. A. Ingles. 2005. Sun exposure, vitamin D receptor gene polymorphisms, and risk of advanced prostate cancer. *Cancer Research* 65 (12):5470–79.

John, E. M., G. G. Schwartz, J. Koo, W. Wang, and S. A. Ingles. 2007. Sun exposure, vitamin D receptor gene polymorphisms, and breast cancer risk in a multiethnic population. *American Journal of Epidemiology* 166:12, doi:10.1093/aje/kwm259.

Judy, W. V., J. H. Hall, W. Dugan, P. D. Toth, and K. Folkers. 1984. Coenzyme Q10 reduction of adriamycin cardiotoxicity. In *Biomedical and clinical aspects of coenzyme Q*, vol. 4, ed. K. Folkers and Y. Yamamura, 231–41. Amsterdam: Elsevier.

Juliano, L. M., and R. R. Griffiths. 2004. A critical review of caffeine withdrawal: Empirical validation of symptoms and signs, incidence, severity, and associated features. *Psychopharmacology* 176 (1):1–29.

Kaaks, R., S. Rinaldi, T. J. Key, F. Berrino, P. H. Peeters, C. Biessy, L. Dossus, A. Lukanova, S. Bingham, K. T. Khaw, N. E. Allen, H. B. Bueno-de-Mesquita, C. H. van Gils, D. Grobbee, H. Boeing, P. H. Lahmann, G. Nagel, J. Chang-Claude, F. Clavel-Chapelon, A. Fournier, A. Thiébaut, C. A. González, J. R. Quirós, M. J. Tormo, E. Ardanaz, P. Amiano, V. Krogh, D. Palli, S. Panico, R. Tumino, P. Vineis, A. Trichopoulou, V. Kalapothaki, D. Trichopoulos, P. Ferrari, T. Norat, R. Saracci, and E. Riboli. 2005. Postmenopausal serum androgens, oestrogens, and breast cancer risk: The European prospective investigation into cancer and nutrition. *Endocrine-Related Cancer* 12 (4):1071–82.

Kalkunte, S., L. Brard, C. O. Granai, and N. Swamy. 2005. Inhibition of angiogenesis by vitamin D-bonding protein: Characterization of anti-endothelial activity of DBP-maf. *Angiogenesis* 8 (4):349–60.

Kara, I. O., B. Sahin, and M. Erkisi. 2006. Palmar-plantar erythrodysesthesia due to docetaxel-capecitabine therapy is treated with vitamin E without dose reduction. *Breast* 15 (3):414–24.

Karin, M., Y. Cao, F. R. Greten, and Z. W. Li. 2002. NF-kappaB in cancer: From innocent bystander to major culprit. *Nature Reviews Cancer* 2 (4):301–10.

Karin, M., and F. R. Greten. 2005. NF-kappaB: Linking inflammation and immunity to cancer development and progression. *Nature Reviews Immunology* 5 (10):749–59.

Karnauchow, P. N. 1995. Melanoma and sun exposure. *Lancet* 346 (8979):915.

Kart, A., M. Elmali, K. Yapar, and H. Yaman. 2008. Occurrence of zeranol in ground beef produced in Kars, Turkey. *Journal of Animal and Veterinary Advances* 7 (5):630–32.

Kasapis, C., and P. D. Thompson. 2005. The effects of physical activity on serum C-reactive protein and inflammatory markers: A systematic review. *Journal of the Americal College of Cardiology* 45 (10):1563–69.

Kawaguchi, Y. 2003. *Effect of AHCC on Gastric Cancer: Kiso and Rinsho*. Tokyo: Life Science Co. Ltd.

Kawamura, N., Y. Kim, and N. Asukai. 2001. Suppression of cellular immunity in men with a past history of posttraumatic stress disorder. *American Journal of Psychiatry* 158 (3):484–86.

Keck, A. S., and J. W. Finley. 2004. Cruciferous vegetables: Cancer protective mechanisms of glucosinolate hydrolysis products and selenium. *Integrative Cancer Therapies* 3 (1):5–12.

Kenner, D. 2001. *AHCC: Active Hexose Correlated Compound*. Salt Lake City, UT: Woodland Publishing.

Kiecolt-Glaser, J. K., M. A. Belury, K. Porter, D. Q. Beversdorf, S. Lemeshow, and R. Glaser. 2007. Depressive symptoms, omega-6:omega-3 fatty acids, and inflammation in older adults. *Psychosomatic Medicine* 69 (3):217–24.

Kihara, T., S. Biro, M. Imamura, S. Yoshifuku, K. Takasaki, Y. Ikeda, Y. Otsuji, S. Minagoe, Y. Toyama, and C. Tei. 2002. Repeated sauna treatment improves vascular endothelial and cardiac function in patients with chronic heart failure. *Journal of the American College of Cardiology* 39 (5):754–59.

Kikuzaki, H., and N. Nakatani. 1993. Antioxidant effects of some ginger constituents. *Journal of Food Science* 58 (6):1407–10.

King, M. C., J. H. Marks, J. B. Mandell; New York Breast Cancer Study Group. 2003. Breast and ovarian cancer risks due to inherited mutations in BRCA1 and BRCA2. *Science* 302 (5645):643–46.

Kirsch, I., B. J. Deacon, T. B. Huedo-Medina, A. Scoboria, T. J. Moore, and B. T. Johnson. 2008. Initial severity and antidepressant benefits: A meta-analysis of data submitted to the Food and Drug Administration. *Public Library of Science (PLoS) Medicine* 5 (2):e45.

Kirsh, V. A., U. Peters, S. T. Mayne, A. F. Subar, N. Chatterjee, C. C. Johnson, R. B. Hayes; Prostate, Lung, Colorectal and Ovarian Cancer Screening Trial. 2007. Prospective study of fruit and vegetable intake and risk of prostate cancer. *Journal of the National Cancer Institute* 99 (15):1200–09.

Kleiman, R., F. R. Earle, W. H. Tallent, and I. A. Wolff. 1970. Retarded hydrolysis by pancreatic lipase of seed oils with trans-3 unsaturation. *Lipids* 5 (6):513–18.

Koebel, C. M., W. Vermi, J. B. Swann, N. Zerafa, S. J. Rodig, L. J. Old, M. J. Smyth, and R. D. Schreiber. 2007. Adaptive immunity maintains occult cancer in an equilibrium state. *Nature* 450:903–07 doi:10.1038/nature06309.

Koga, C., K. Itoh, M. Aoki, Y. Suefuji, M. Yoshida, S. Asosina, K. Esaki, and T. Kameyama. 2001. Anxiety and pain suppress the natural killer cell activity in oral surgery outpatients. *Journal of Oral Surgery, Oral Medicine, Oral Pathology, Oral Radiology, and Endodontics* 91 (6):654–58.

Kogon, M. M., A. Biswas, D. Pearl, R. W. Carlson, and D. Spiegel. 1997. Effects of medical and psychotherapeutic treatment on the survival of women with metastatic breast carcinoma. *Cancer* 80 (2):225–30.

Kolata, G., and A. Pollack. 2008. Costly cancer drug offers hope, but also a dilemma. *New York Times*, July 6, Health section.

Kolb, N., L. Vallorani, N. Milanovic, and V. Stocchi. 2004. Evaluation of marine algae wakame (Undaria *pinnatifida*) and kombu (*Laminaria digitata japonica*) as food supplements. *Food Technology and Biotechnology* 42 (1):57–61.

Kösters, J. P., and P. C. Gøtzsche. 2003. Regular self-examination or clinical examination for early detection of breast cancer. *Cochrane Database of Systematic Reviews* 2, no. CD003373, doi:10.1002/14651858.CD003373.

Kozlovsky, A. S., P. B. Moser, S. Reiser, and R. A. Anderson. 1986. Effects of diets high in simple sugars on urinary chromium losses. *Metabolism* 35 (6):515–18.

Kraft, J., J. K. G. Kramer, F. Schoene, J. R. Chambers, and G. Jahreis. 2008. Extensive analysis of long-chain polyunsaturated fatty acids, CLA, trans-18:1 isomers, and plasmalogenic lipids in different retail beef types. *Journal of Agricultural and Food Chemistry* 56 (12):4775–82.

Kromann, N., and A. Green. 1980. Epidemiological studies in the Upernavik district, Greenland: Incidence of some chronic diseases 1950–1974. *Acta medica Scandinavia* 208 (5):401–06.

Kundi, M., K. Mild, L. Hardell, and M. O. Mattsson. 2004. Mobile telephones and cancer: A review of epidemiological evidence. *Journal of Toxicology and Environmental Health B: Critical Reviews* 7 (5):351–84.

Kusaka, Y., H. Kondou, and K. Morimoto. 1992. Healthy lifestyles are associated with higher natural killer cell activity. *Preventive Medicine* 21 (5):602–15.

Labbate, L. A. 1999. Sex and serotonin reuptake inhibitor antidepressants. *Psychiatric Annals* 29:571–79.

Labrecque, L., S. Lamy, A. Chapus, S. Mihoubi, Y. Durocher, B. Cass, M. W. Bojanowski, D. Gingras, and R. Béliveau. 2005. Combined inhibition of PDGF and VEGF receptors by ellagic acid, a dietary-derived phenolic compound. *Carcinogenesis* 26 (4):821–26.

Lane, J. D., J. E. Seskevich, and C. F. Pieper. 2007. Brief meditation training can improve perceived stress and negative mood. *Alternative Therapies in Health and Medicine* 13 (1):38–44.

LaPerriere, A. R., M. H. Antoni, N. Schneiderman, G. Ironson, N. Klimas, P. Caralis, and M. A. Fletcher. 1990. Exercise intervention attenuates emotional distress and natural killer cell decrements following notification of positive serologic status for HIV-1. *Biofeedback and Self-Regulation* 15 (3):229–42.

Larsen, T. M., S. Toubro, and A. Astrup. 2003. Efficacy and safety of dietary supplements containing conjugated linoleic acid (CLA) for the treatment of obesity: Evidence from animal and human studies. *Journal of Lipid Research* 44 (12):2234–41.

Larsson, S. C., E. Giovannucci, and A. Wolk. 2004. Dietary folate intake and incidence of ovarian cancer: The Swedish Mammography Cohort. *Journal of the National Cancer Institute* 96 (5):396–402.

Latenkov, V. P. 1985. Circadian rhythms of adrenaline and noradrenaline excretion in man in normal conditions and after alcohol intake. [In Russian.] *Biulleten' eksperimental'noi biologii i meditsiny (Bulletin of Experimental Biology and Medicine)* 99 (3):346–48.

Laubmeier, K. K., S. G. Zakowski, and J. P. Bair. 2004. The role of spirituality in the psychological adjustment to cancer: A test of the transactional model of stress and coping. *International Journal of Behavioral Medicine* 11 (1):48–55.

Lawson, L. D., and Z. J. Wang. 2001. Low allicin release from garlic supplements: A major problem due to the sensitivities of alliinase activity. *Journal of Agricultural and Food Chemistry* 49 (5):2592–99.

Leaf, C. 2004. Why we're losing the war on cancer (and how to win it). *Fortune* 149 (6):76–97.

Leclercq, I. A., G. C. Farrell, C. Sempoux, A. dela Peña, and Y. Horsmans. 2004. Curcumin inhibits NF-kappaB activation and reduces the severity of experimental steatohepatitis in mice. *Journal of Hepatology* 41 (6):926–34.

Lee, A. T., and A. Cerami. 1992. Role of glycation in aging. *Annals of the New York Academy of Sciences* 663:63–70.

Lee, Y. S., I. S. Chung, I. R. Lee, K. H. Kim, W. S. Hong, and Y. S. Yun. 1997. Activation of multiple effector pathways of immune system by the antineoplastic immunostimulator acidic polysaccharide ginsan isolated from Panax ginseng. *Anticancer Research* 17 (1A):323–31.

Leipner, J., and R. Saller. 2000. Systemic enzyme therapy in oncology: Effect and mode of action. *Drugs* 59 (4):769–80.

Lemann, J. 1976. Evidence that glucose ingestion inhibits net renal tubular reabsorption of calcium and magnesium. *Journal of Clinical Nutrition* 70:236–45.

Le Marchand, L., S. P. Murphy, J. H. Hankin, L. R. Wilkens, and L. N. Kolonel. 2000. Intake of flavonoids and lung cancer. *Journal of the National Cancer Institute* 92 (2):154–60.

Lenoir, M., F. Serre, L. Cantin, and S. H. Ahmed. 2007. Intense sweetness surpasses cocaine reward. *PLoS ONE* 2 (1):e698.

LeShan, L. 1999. *Cancer As a Turning Point: A Handbook for People with Cancer, Their Families, and Health Professionals.* New York: Plume-Penguin.

Leung, P. S., W. J. Aronson, T. H. Ngo, L. A. Golding, and R. J. Barnard. 2004. Exercise alters the IGF axis *in vivo* and increases p53 protein in prostate tumor cells *in vitro. Journal of Applied Physiology* 96 (2):450–54.

Levine, M. E., M. Gillis, S. Yanchis, C. Voss, R. M. Stern, and K. L. Koch. 2006. Protein and ginger for the treatment of chemotherapy-induced delayed nausea and gastric dysrhythmia. *Neurogastroenterology and Motility* 18 (6):488.

Levine, P. A. 1997. *Waking the Tiger: Healing Trauma—The Innate Capacity to Transform Overwhelming Experiences.* Berkeley, CA: North Atlantic Books.

Levy, S., R. Herberman, M. Lippman, and T. d'Angelo. 1987. Correlation of stress factors with sustained depression of natural killer cell activity and predicted prognosis in patients with breast cancer. *Journal of Clinical Oncology* 5 (3):348–53.

Levy, S. M., R. B. Herberman, A. M. Maluish, B. Schlien, and M. Lippman. 1985. Prognostic risk assessment in primary breast cancer by behavioral and immunological parameters. *Health Psychology* 4 (2):99–113.

Li, Y., C. Xu, Q. Zhang, J. Y. Liu, and R. X. Tan. 2005. In vitro anti-Helicobacter pylori action of 30 Chinese herbal medicines used to treat ulcer diseases. *Journal of Ethnopharmacology* 98 (3):329–33.

Lin, J., J. E. Manson, I. M. Lee, N. R. Cook, J. E. Buring, and S. M. Zhang. 2007. Intakes of calcium and vitamin D and breast cancer risk in women. *Archives of Internal Medicine* 167 (10):1050–59.

Lockwood, K., S. Moesgaard, and K. Folkers. 1994. Partial and complete regression of breast cancer in patients in relation to dosage of coenzyme Q10. *Biochemical and Biophysical Research Communications* 199 (3):1504–08.

Lockwood, K., S. Moesgaard, T. Hanioka, and K. Folkers. 1994. Apparent partial remission of breast cancer in "high risk" patients supplemented with nutritional antioxidants, essential fatty acids, and coenzyme $Q_{10}$. *Molecular Aspects of Medicine* 15 Suppl.:S231–40.

Lopez, A. M., L. Wallace, R. T. Dorr, M. Koff, E. M. Hersh, and D. S. Alberts. 1999. Topical DMSO treatment for pegylated liposomal doxorubicin-induced palmar-plantar erythrodysesthesia. *Cancer Chemotherapy and Pharmacology* 44 (4):303–06.

Lopez, I., C. Goudou, V. Ribrag, C. Sauvage, G. Hazebroucq, and F. Dreyfus. 1994. Treatment of mucositis with vitamin E during administration of neutropenic antineoplastic agents. [In French.] *Annales de médecine interne* 145 (6):405–08.

Lopez-Garcia, E., M. B. Schulze, J. B. Meigs, J. E. Manson, N. Rifai, M. J. Stampfer, W. C. Willett, and F. B. Hu. 2005. Consumption of trans fatty acids is related to plasma biomarkers of inflammation and endothelial dysfunction. *Journal of Nutrition* 135 (3):562–66.

Lutz, A., L. L. Greischar, N. B. Rawlings, M. Ricard, and R. J. Davidson. 2004. Long-term meditators self-induce high-amplitude gamma synchrony during mental practice. *Proceedings of the National Academy of Sciences* 101 (46):16,369–73.

Machado Rocha, F. C., S. C. Stéfano, H. R. De Cássia, L. M. Rosa Oliveira, and D. X. Da Silveira. 2008. Therapeutic use of Cannabis sativa on chemotherapy-induced nausea and vomiting among cancer patients: Systematic review and meta-analysis. *European Journal of Cancer Care* 17 (5):431–43.

Manna, S. K., A. Mukhopadhyay, and B. B. Aggarwal. 2000. Resveratrol suppresses TNF-induced activation of nuclear transcription factors NF-kappa B, activator protein-1, and apoptosis: Potential role of reactive oxygen intermediates and lipid peroxidation. *Journal of Immunology* 164 (12):6509–19.

Marcsek, Z., Z. Kocsis, M. Jakab, B. Szende, and A. Tompa. 2004. The efficacy of tamoxifen in estrogen receptor–positive breast cancer cells is enhanced by a medical nutriment. *Cancer Biotherapy and Radiopharmaceuticals* 19 (6):746–53.

Marks, L. S., Y. Fradet, I. L. Deras, A. Blase, J. Mathis, S. M. Aubin, A. T. Cancio, M. Desaulniers, W. J. Ellis, H. Rittenhouse, and J. Groskopf. 2007. PCA3 molecular urine assay for prostate cancer in men undergoing repeat biopsy. *Urology* 69 (3):532–35.

Maruyama, H., H. Tamauchi, M. Hashimoto, and T. Nakano. 2003. Antitumor activity and immune response of Mekabu fucoidan extracted from Sporophyll of *Undaria pinnatifida*. *In Vivo* 17 (3):245–49.

Marx, J. 2004. Cancer research: Inflammation and cancer—The link grows stronger. *Science* 306 (5698):966–68.

Matsui, Y., J. Uhara, S. Satoi, M. Kaibori, H. Yamada, H. Kitade, A. Imamura, S. Takai, Y. Kawaguchi, A. H. Kwon, and Y. Kamiyama. 2002. Improved prognosis of postoperative hepatocellular carcinoma patients when treated with functional foods: A prospective cohort study. *Journal of Hepatology* 37 (1):78–86.

McClain, J., S. Clipp, J. Hoffman-Bolton, K. Helzlsouer, and K. Visvanathan. 2008. Association between physical activity, sleep duration, and cancer risk among women in Washington County, MD: A prospective cohort study. Abstract. *Cancer Prevention Research* 1 (7 Suppl.):B145, doi:10.1158/1940-6207.PREV-08-B145.

McCulloch, M., T. Jezierski, M. Broffman, A. Hubbard, K. Turner, and T. Janecki. 2006a. Diagnostic accuracy of canine scent detection in early- and late-stage lung and breast cancers. *Integrative Cancer Therapies* 5 (1):30–39.

McCulloch, M., C. See, X. J. Shu, M. Broffman, A. Kramer, W. Y. Fan, J. Gao, W. Lieb, K. Shieh, and J. M. Colford, Jr. 2006b. Astragalus-based Chinese herbs and platinum-based chemotherapy for advanced non-small-cell lung cancer: Meta-analysis of randomized trials. *Journal of Clinical Oncology* 24 (3):419–30.

McTiernan, A., C. Kooperberg, E. White, S. Wilcox, R. Coates, L. L. Adams-Campbell, N. Woods, and J. Ockene; Women's Health Initiative Cohort Study. 2003. Recreational physical activity and the risk of breast cancer in postmenopausal women: The Women's Health Initiative Cohort Study. *Journal of the American Medical Association* 290 (10):1331–36.

Meares, A. 1978. Regression of osteogenic sarcoma metastases associated with intensive meditation. *Medical Journal of Australia* 2 (9):433.

Metcalf, N. 2004. Drugs vs. talk therapy: 3,079 readers rate their care for depression and anxiety. *Consumer Reports*, October, 22–29.

Meyer, F., I. Bairati, A. Fortin, M. Gélinas, N. Abdenour, F. Brochet, and B. Têtu. 2008. Interaction between antioxidant vitamin supplementation and cigarette smoking during radiation therapy in relation to long-term effects on recurrrence and mortality: A randomized trial among head and neck cancer patients. *International Journal of Cancer* 122 (7):1679–83.

Meyerhardt, J. A., D. Heseltine, D. Niedzwiecki, D. Hollis, L. B. Saltz, R. J. Mayer, J. Thomas, H. Nelson, R. Whittom, A. Hantel, R. L. Schilsky, and C. S. Fuchs. 2006. Impact of physical activity on cancer recurrence and survival in patients with stage III colon cancer: Findings from CALGB 89803. *Journal of Clinical Oncology* 24 (22):3535–41.

Michaud, D. S., K. Joshipura, E. Giovannucci, and C. S. Fuchs. 2007. A prospective study of periodontal disease and pancreatic cancer in US male health professionals. *Journal of the National Cancer Institute* 99 (2):1–5.

Michaud, D. S., S. Liu, E. Giovannucci, W. C. Willett, G. A. Colditz, and C. S. Fuchs. 2002. Dietary sugar, glycemic load, and pancreatic cancer risk in a prospective study. *Journal of the National Cancer Institute* 94 (17):1293–1300.

Miner, J. L., C. A. Cederberg, M. K. Nielsen, X. Chen, and C. A. Baile. 2001. Conjugated linoleic acid (CLA), body fat, and apoptosis. *Obesity Research* 9 (2):129–34.

Miniño, A. M., M. P. Heron, S. L. Murphy, and K. D. Kochanek; Centers for Disease Control and Prevention National Center for Health Statistics National Vital Statistics System. 2007. Deaths: Final data for 2004. *National Vital Statistics Reports* 55 (19):1–119.

Moertel, C. G., T. R. Fleming, E. T. Creagan, J. Rubin, M. J. O'Connell, and M. M. Ames. 1985. High-dose vitamin C versus placebo in the treatment of patients with advanced cancer who have had no prior chemotherapy: A randomized double-blind comparison. *New England Journal of Medicine* 312 (3):137–41.

Moffat, L., E. Cameron, and A. Campbell. 1983. High-dose ascorbate therapy and cancer. In *Protective agents in cancer*, ed. D. C. H. McBrien, and T. F. Slater, 243–56. New York: Academic Press.

Mohan, R., J. Sivak, P. Ashton, L. A. Russo, B. Q. Pham, N. Kasahara, M. B. Raizman, and M. E. Fini. 2000. Curcuminoids inhibit the angiogenic response stimulated by fibroblast growth factor-2, including expression of matrix metalloproteinase gelatinase B. *Journal of Biological Chemistry* 275 (14):10405–12.

Morgan, A. G., W. A. F. McAdam, C. Pacsoo, and A. Darnborough. 1982. Comparison between cimetidine and Caved-S in the treatment of gastric ulceration, and subsequent maintenance therapy. *Gut* 23 (6):545–51.

Morgan, N. P., K. D. Graves, E. A. Poggi, and B. D. Cheson. 2008. Implementing an expressive writing study in a cancer clinic. *Oncologist* 13 (2):196–204.

Morris, M. S., and R. S. Knorr. 1996. Adult leukemia and proximity-based surrogates for exposure to Pilgrim plant's nuclear emissions. *Archives of Environmental Health* 51 (4):266–74.

Moss, R. W. 2000. *Antioxidants Against Cancer*. Brooklyn, NY: Equinox Press.

Moss, R. W. 2004. Losing the war on cancer. *Townsend Letter for Doctors and Patients* 251:33.

Mozaffarian, D., M. B. Katan, A. Ascherio, M. J. Stampfer, and W. C. Willett. 2006. Trans-fatty acids and cardiovascular disease. *New England Journal of Medicine* 354 (15):1601–13.

Muckle, G., P. Ayotte, E. Dewailly, S. W. Jacobson, and J. L. Jacobson. 2001. Determinants of polychlorinated biphenyls and methylmercury exposure in Inuit women of childbearing age. *Environmental Health Perspectives* 109 (9):957–63.

Mulhall, B. P., G. R. Veerappan, and J. L. Jackson. 2005. Meta-analysis: Computed tomographic colonography. *Annals of Internal Medicine* 142 (8):635–50.

Murata, A., F. Morishige, and H. Yamaguchi. 1982. Prolongation of survival times of terminal cancer patients by administration of large doses of ascorbate. *International Journal for Vitamin and Nutrition Research Supplement* 23:103–13.

Muscaritoli, M., M. Bossola, Z. Aversa, R. Bellantone, and F. Rossi Fanelli. 2006. Prevention and treatment of cancer cachexia: New insights into an old problem. *European Journal of Cancer* 42 (1):31–41.

Nagabhushan, M., and S. V. Bhide. 1992. Curcumin as an inhibitor of cancer. *Journal of the American College of Nutrition* 11 (2):192–8.

Nair, M. P., Z. A. Kronfol, and S. A. Schwartz. 1990. Effects of alcohol and nicotine on cytotoxic functions of human lymphocytes. *Clinical Immunology and Immunopathology* 54 (3):395–409.

Nandave, M., I. Mohanty, T. C. Nag, S. K. Ojha, R. Mittal, S. Kumari, and D. S. Arya. 2007. Cardioprotective response to chronic administration of vitamin E in isoproterenol induced myocardial necrosis: Hemodynamic, biochemical, and ultrastructural studies. *Indian Journal of Clinical Biochemistry* 22 (1):22–28.

National Academy of Sciences. 1982. *Diet, Nutrition, and Cancer*. Washington, DC: National Academy Press.

National Cancer Institute. 2007. FactSheet: Screening mammograms—Questions and answers. www.cancer.gov/cancertopics/factsheet/detection/screening-mammograms (accessed March 9, 2009).

———. 2008. Hydrazine sulfate (PDQ): Human/clinical studies. www.cancer.gov/cancertopics/pdq/cam/hydrazinesulfate/HealthProfessional/page6 (accessed May 16, 2009).

National Center on Physical Activity and Disability. 2009. Disability/Condition: Cancer and Exercise—Indications for the Termination of Testing or Training. www.ncpad.org/disability/fact_sheet.php?sheet=195&section=1451.

Naurath, H. J., E. Joosten, R. Riezler, S. P. Stabler, R. H. Allen, and J. Lindenbaum. 1995. Effects of vitamin B12, folate, and vitamin B6 supplements in elderly people with normal serum vitamin concentrations. *Lancet* 346 (8967):85–9.

Nelson, A. N., and J. H. Haig. 1997. *The New Nelson Japanese-English Character Dictionary*. Rev. ed. Rutland, VT: Tuttle Publishing.

Nelson, J. E., and R. E. Harris. 2000. Inverse association of prostate cancer and non-steroidal anti-inflammatory drugs (NSAIDs): Results of a case-control study. *Oncology Reports* 7 (1):169–70.

Nicolson, G. L. 2005. Lipid replacement/antioxidant therapy as an adjunct supplement to reduce the adverse effects of cancer therapy and restore mitochondrial function. *Pathology and Oncology Research* 11 (3):139–44.

Nielsen, O. S., M. Horsman, and J. Overgaard. 2001. A future for hyperthermia in cancer treatment? *European Journal of Cancer* 37 (13):1587–89.

Null, G., H. Robins, M. Tanenbaum, and P. Jennings. 1997. Vitamin C and treatment of cancer: Part I—Abstracts and commentary from the scientific literature. *Townsend Letter for Doctors and Patients*, May. www.garynull.com/documents/vitaminc%2Dcancer.htm.

Nurnberger, Jr., J. I., and L. J. Bierut. 2007. Seeking the connections: Alcoholism and our genes. *Scientific American* 296 (4):46–53.

Office of the Surgeon General. 1990. *The Health Benefits of Smoking Cessation: A Report of the Surgeon General.* Centers for Disease Control and Prevention (CDC), Office on Smoking and Health. http://profiles.nlm.nih.gov/NN/B/B/C/T.

O'Keefe, S., S. Gaskins-Wright, V. Wiley, and I. Chen. 1994. Levels of trans geometrical isomers of essential fatty acids in some unhydrogenated US vegetable oils. *Journal of Food Lipids* 1 (3):165–76.

Okuno, M., K. Kajiwara, S. Imai, T. Kobayashi, N. Honma, T. Maki, K. Suruga, T. Goda, S. Takase, Y. Muto, and H. Moriwaki. 1997. Perilla oil prevents the excessive growth of visceral adipose tissue in rats by down-regulating adipocyte differentiation. *Journal of Nutrition* 127 (9):1752–57.

Olsen, O., and P. C. Gøtzsche. 2001. Cochrane review on screening for breast cancer with mammography. *Lancet* 358 (9290):1340–42.

Omenn, G. S., G. Goodman, M. Thornquist, J. Grizzle, L. Rosenstock, S. Barnhart, J. Balmes, M. G. Cherniack, M. R. Cullen, and A. Glass. 1994. The beta-carotene and retinol efficacy trial (CARET) for chemoprevention of lung cancer in high-risk populations: Smokers and asbestos-exposed workers. *Cancer Research* 54 (Suppl. 7):2038S–43.

O'Neal, D. P., L. R. Hirsch, N. J. Halas, J. D. Payne, and J. L. West. 2004. Photo-thermal tumor ablation in mice using near infrared-absorbing nanoparticles. *Cancer Letters* 209 (2):171–76.

Ooi, V. E., and F. Liu. 2000. Immunomodulation and anti-cancer activity of polysaccharide-protein complexes. *Current Medicinal Chemistry* 7 (7):715–29.

O'Reilly, M. S., L. Holmgren, Y. Shing, C. Chen, R. A. Rosenthal, M. Moses, W. S. Lane, Y. Cao, E. H. Sage, and J. Folkman. 1994. Angiostatin: A novel angiogenesis inhibitor that mediates the suppression of metastases by a Lewis lung carcinoma. *Cell* 79 (2):315–28.

Orel, S. G., and M. D. Schnall. 2001. MR Imaging of the breast for the detection, diagnosis, and staging of breast cancer. *Radiology* 220 (1):13–30.

Ornish, D., M. J. Magbanua, G. Weidner, V. Weinberg, C. Kemp, C. Green, M. D. Mattie, R. Marlin, J. Simko, K. Shinohara, C. M. Haqq, and P. R. Carroll. 2008. Changes in prostate gene expression in men undergoing an intensive nutrition and lifestyle intervention. *Proceedings of the National Academy of Sciences* 105 (24):8369–74.

Ornish, D., G. Weidner, W. R. Fair, R. Marlin, E. B. Pettengill, C. J. Raisin, S. Dunn-Emke, L. Crutchfield, F. N. Jacobs, R. J. Barnard, W. J. Aronson, P. McCormac, D. J. McKnight, J. D. Fein, A. M. Dnistrian, J. Weinstein, T. H. Ngo, N. R. Mendell, and P. R. Carroll. 2005. Intensive lifestyle changes may affect the progression of prostate cancer. *Journal of Urology* 174 (3):1065–69.

Owen, N., and A. Steptoe. 2003. Natural killer cell and proinflammatory cytokine responses to mental stress: Associations with heart rate and heart rate variability. *Biological Psychology* 63 (2):101–15.

Oztasan, N., S. Taysi, K. Gumustekin, K. Altinkaynak, O. Aktas, H. Timur, E. Siktar, S. Keles, S. Akar, F. Akcay, S. Dane, and M. Gul. 2004. Endurance training attenuates exercise-induced oxidative stress in erythrocytes in rat. *European Journal of Applied Physiology* 91 (5–6):622–27.

Pace, T. W., T. C. Mletzko, O. Alagbe, D. L. Musselman, C. B. Nemeroff, A. H. Miller, and C. M. Heim. 2006. Increased stress-induced inflammatory responses in male patients with major depression and increased early life stress. *American Journal of Psychiatry* 163 (9):1630–33.

Packer, L., K. Kraemer, and G. Rimbach. 2001. Molecular aspects of lipoic acid in the prevention of diabetes complications. *Nutrition* 17 (10):888–95.

Padayatty, S. J., H. D. Riordan, S. M. Hewitt, A. Katz, L. J. Hoffer, and M. Levine. 2006. Intravenously administered vitamin C as cancer therapy: Three cases. *Canadian Medical Association Journal* 174 (7):937–42.

Padayatty, S. J., H. Sun, Y. Wang, H. D. Riordan, S. M. Hewitt, A. Katz, R. A. Wesley, and M. Levine. 2004. Vitamin C pharmacokinetics: Implications for oral and intravenous use. *Annals of Internal Medicine* 140 (7):533–37.

Pantuck, A. J., J. T. Leppert, N. Zomorodian, W. Aronson, J. Hong, R. J. Barnard, N. Seeram, H. Liker, H. Wang, R. Elashoff, D. Heber, M. Aviram, L. Ignarro, and A. Belldegrun. 2006. Phase II study of pomegranate juice for men with rising prostate-specific antigen following surgery or radiation for prostate cancer. *Clinical Cancer Research* 12 (13):4018–26.

Pasteur, L. 1858. Memoire sur la fermentation appelle lactique. Annales de chimie et de physique 3ème série 52:404–18.

Patel, A. V., E. E. Callel, L. Bernstein, A. H. Wu, and M. J. Thun. 2003. Recreational physical activity and risk of postmenopausal breast cancer in a large cohort of U.S. women. *Cancer Causes and Control* 14 (6):519–29.

Patel, A. V., C. Rodriguez, E. J. Jacobs, L. Solomon, M. J. Thun, and E. E. Calle. 2005. Recreational physical activity and risk of prostate cancer in a large cohort of U.S. men. *Cancer Epidemiology, Biomarkers, and Prevention* 14 (1):275–79.

Patel, M., F. Gutzwiller, F. Paccaud, and A. Marazzi. 1989. A meta-analysis of acupuncture for chronic pain. *International Journal of Epidemiology* 18 (4):900–06.

Pathak, A. K., M. Bhutani, R. Guleria, S. Bal, A. Mohan, B. K. Mohanti, A. Sharma, R. Pathak, N. K. Bhardwaj, K. N. Prasad, and V. Kochupillai. 2005. Chemotherapy alone vs. chemotherapy plus high-dose multiple antioxidants in patients with advanced non small cell lung cancer. *Journal of the American College of Nutrition* 24 (1):16–21.

Paul-Labrador, M., D. Polk, J. H. Dwyer, I. Velasquez, S. Nidich, M. Rainforth, R. Schneider, and C. N. Merz. 2006. Effects of a randomized controlled trial of transcendental meditation on components of the metabolic syndrome in subjects with coronary heart disease. *Archives of Internal Medicine* 166 (11):1218–24.

Pearsall, P. 2007. In awe of the heart. *Alternative Therapies in Health and Medicine* 13 (4):16–19.

Penedo, F. J., and J. R. Dahn. 2005. Exercise and well-being: A review of mental and physical health benefits associated with physical activity. *Current Opinion in Psychiatry* 18 (2):189–93.

Penn, M. S., and E. E. Bakken. 2007. Heart-brain medicine: Where we go from here and why. *Cleveland Clinic Journal of Medicine* 74 (Suppl. 1):S4–6.

Pert, C. B. 1999. *Molecules of Emotion: Why You Feel the Way You Feel.* New York: Simon and Schuster.

Peto, R., R. Doll, J. D. Buckley, and M. B. Sporn. 1981. Can dietary beta-carotene materially reduce human cancer rates? *Nature* 290 (5803):201–08.

Petrakis, N. L., and M. C. King. 1976. Genetic markers and cancer epidemiology. *Cancer* 39 (54):1861–66.

Piyathilake, C. J., M. Macaluso, I. Brill, D. C. Heimburger, and E. E. Partridge. 2007. Lower red blood cell folate enhances the HPV-16-associated risk of cervical intraepithelial neoplasia. *Nutrition* 23 (3):203–10.

Potter, J. D., and A. J. McMichael. 1986. Diet and cancer of the colon and rectum: A case-control study. Journal of the National Cancer Institute 76 (4):557–69.

Prasad, A. S. 1998. Zinc and immunity. *Molecular and Cellular Biochemistry* 188 (1–2):63–69.

Prasad, K. N., W. C. Cole, B. Kumar, and K. C. Prasad. 2001. Scientific rationale for using high-dose multiple micronutrients as an adjunct to standard and experimental cancer therapies. *Journal of the American College of Nutrition* 20 (Suppl. 5):450S–63.

Prasad, K. N., A. Kumar, V. Kochupillai, and W. C. Cole. 1999. High doses of multiple antioxidant vitamins: Essential ingredients in improving the efficacy of standard cancer therapy. *Journal of the American College of Nutrition* 18 (1):13–25.

Pratap, A., and P. C. Schroy III. 2007. Physical activity and colorectal cancer survival: The more METS the better. *Gastroenterology* 132 (1):456–58.

Premkumar, V. G., S. Yuvaraj, K. Vijayasarathy, S. Gangadaran, and P. Sachdanandam. 2007. Effect of coenzyme $Q_{10}$, riboflavin, and niacin on serum CEA and CA 15-3 levels in breast cancer patients undergoing tamoxifen therapy. *Biological and Pharmaceutical Bulletin* 30 (2):367–70.

Price, M. A., C. C. Tennant, P. N. Butow, R. C. Smith, S. J. Kennedy, M. B. Kossoff, and S. M. Dunn. 2001. The role of psychosocial factors in the development of breast carcinoma: Part II—Life event stressors, social support, defense style, and emotional control and their interactions. *Cancer* 91 (4):686–97.

Pugliese, P. T., K. Jordan, H. Cederberg, and J. Brohult. 1998. Some biological actions of alkylglycerols from shark liver oil. *Journal of Alternative and Complementary Medicine* 4 (1):87–99.

Puri, A., S. K. Maulik, R. Ray, and V. Bhatnagar. 2001. Cardioprotective effect of vitamin E in doxorubicin induced acute cardiotoxicity in rats. *Journal of Indian Association of Pediatric Surgeons* 6 (4):112–8.

Quartana, P. J., K. K. Laubmeier, and S. G. Zakowski. 2006. Psychological adjustment following diagnosis and treatment of cancer: An examination of the moderating role of positive and negative emotional expressivity. *Journal of Behavioral Medicine* 29 (5):487–98.

Rahman, K. M., Y. Li, and F. H. Sarkar. 2004. Inactivation of akt and NF-kappaB play important roles during indole 3-carbinol-induced apoptosis in breast cancer cells. *Nutrition and Cancer* 48 (1):84–94.

Rajpathak, S. N., A. P. McGinn, H. D. Strickler, T. E. Rohan, M. Pollak, A. R. Cappola, L. Kuller, X. N. Xue, A. B. Newman, E. S. Strotmeyer, B. M. Psaty, and R. C. Kaplan. 2008. Insulin-like growth factor-(IGF)-axis, inflammation, and glucose intolerance among older adults. *Growth Hormone and IGF Research* 18 (2):166–73.

Rea, W. J., Y. Pan, A. R. Johnson, G. H. Ross, H. E. Suyama, and E. J. Fenyves. 1996. Reduction of chemical sensitivity by means of depuration, physical therapy, and nutritional supplementation in a controlled environment. *Journal of Nutritional and Environmental Medicine* 6 (2):141–48.

Reiche, E. M., S. O. Nunes, and H. K. Morimoto. 2004. Stress, depression, the immune system, and cancer. *Lancet Oncology* 5 (10):617–25.

Renehan, A. G., M. Tyson, M. Egger, R. F. Heller, and M. Zwahlen. 2008. Body-mass index and incidence of cancer: A systematic review and meta-analysis of prospective observational studies. *Lancet* 371 (9612):569–78.

Rhodes, R. 1986. *The Making of the Atomic Bomb.* New York: Simon and Schuster.

Richardson, M. A., T. Sanders, J. L. Palmer, A. Greisinger, and S. E. Singletary. 2000. Complementary/alternative medicine use in a comprehensive cancer center and the implications for oncology. *Journal of Clinical Oncology* 18 (13):2505–14.

Ries, L. A. G., M. P. Eisner, C. L. Kosary, B. F. Hankey, B. A. Miller, L. Clegg, B. K. Edwards, eds. 2002. *SEER Cancer Statistics Review, 1973–1999.* Bethesda, MD: National Cancer Institute. http://seer.cancer.gov/csr/1973_1999/index.html.

Riordan, N., J. Jackson, and H. D. Riordan. 1996. Intravenous vitamin C in a terminal cancer patient. *Journal of Orthomolecular Medicine* 11 (2):80–82.

Roehm, D. 1983. Effects of a program of sauna baths and megavitamins on adipose DDE and PCBs and on clearing of symptoms of Agent Orange (dioxin) toxicity. *Clinical Research* 31 (2):243A.

Rogers, S. A. 2002. *Detoxify or Die.* Sarasota, FL: Prestige Pubs.

Rooprai, H. K., A. Kandanearatchi, S. L. Maidment, M. Christidou, G. Trillo-Pazos, D. T. Dexter, G. Rucklidge, W. Widmer, and G. J. Pilkington. 2001. Evaluation of the effects of swainsonine, captopril, tangeretin, and nobiletin on the biological behaviour of brain tumour cells in vitro. *Neuropathology and Applied Neurobiology* 27 (1):29–39.

Rossouw, J. E., G. L. Anderson, R. L. Prentice, A. Z. LaCroix, C. Kooperberg, M. L. Stefanick, R. D. Jackson, S. A. Beresford, B. V. Howard, K. C. Johnson, J. M. Kotchen, J. Ockene; Writing Group for the Women's Health Initiative Investigators. 2002. Risks and benefits of estrogen plus progestin in healthy postmenopausal women: Principal results from the Women's Health Initiative randomized controlled trial. *Journal of the American Medical Association* 288 (3):321–33.

Sadetzki, S., A. Chetrit, A. Jarus-Hakak, E. Cardis, Y. Deutch, S. Duvdevani, A. Zultan, I. Novikov, L. Freedman, and M. Wolf. 2008. Cellular phone use and risk of benign and malignant parotid gland tumors: A nationwide case-control study. *American Journal of Epidemiology* 167 (4):457–67.

Sahakian, A., and W. H. Frishman. 2007. Humor and the cardiovascular system. *Alternative Therapies in Health and Medicine* 13 (4):56–58.

Sakalová, A., P. R. Bock, L. Dedík, J. Hanisch, W. Schiess, S. Gazová, I. Chabronová, D. Holomanova, M. Mistrík, and M. Hrubisko. 2001. Retrolective cohort study of an additive therapy with an oral enzyme preparation in patients with multiple myeloma. *Cancer Chemotherapy and Pharmacology* 47 Suppl.:S38–44.

Sandlund, E. S., and T. Norlander. 2000. The effects of tai chi chuan relaxation and exercise on stress responses and well-being: An overview of research. *International Journal of Stress Management* 7 (2):139–49.

Schernhammer, E. S., F. Berrino, V. Krogh, G. Secreto, A. Micheli, E. Venturelli, S. Sieri, C. T. Sempos, A. Cavalleri, H. J. Schünemann, S. Strano, and P. Muti. 2008. Urinary 6-sulfatoxymelatonin levels and risk of breast cancer in postmenopausal women. *Journal of the National Cancer Institute* 100 (12):898–905.

Schernhammer, E. S., F. Laden, F. E. Speizer, W. C. Willett, D. J. Hunter, I. Kawachi, and G. A. Colditz. 2001. Rotating night shifts and risk of breast cancer in women participating in the Nurses' Health Study. *Journal of the National Cancer Institute* 93 (20):1563–68.

Schernhammer, E. S., F. Laden, F. E. Speizer, W. C. Willett, D. J. Hunter, I. Kawachi, C. S. Fuchs, and G. A. Colditz. 2003. Night-shift work and risk of colorectal cancer in the Nurses' Health Study. *Journal of the National Cancer Institute* 95 (11):825–28.

Schnare, D. W., M. Ben, and M. G. Shields. 1984. Body burden reductions of PCBs, PBBs, and chlorinated pesticides in human subjects. *AMBIO, a Journal of the Human Environment* 13 (5–6):378–80.

Schnare, D. W., and P. C. Robinson. 1986. Reduction of the human body burdens of hexachlorobenzene and polychlorinated biphenyls. *IRAC Scientific Publications* 77:597–603.

Schwenke, D. C. 2002. Does lack of tocopherols and tocotrienols put women at increased risk of breast cancer? *Journal of Nutritional Biochemistry* 13 (1):2–20.

Scientific Committee on Veterinary Measures Relating to Public Health. 1999. Assessment of potential risks to human health from hormone residues in bovine meat and meat products. European Commission Directorate-General XXIV Consumer Policy and Consumer Health Protection XXIV/B3/SC4.

Seeram, N. P., L. S. Adams, Y. Zhang, R. Lee, D. Sand, H. S. Scheuller, and D. Heber. 2006. Blackberry, black raspberry, blueberry, cranberry, red raspberry, and strawberry extracts inhibit growth and stimulate apoptosis in human cancer cells in vitro. *Journal of Agricultural and Food Chemistry* 54 (25):9329–39.

Sephton, S., and D. Spiegel. 2003. Circadian disruption in cancer: A neuroendocrine-immune pathway from stress to disease? *Brain Behavior, and Immunity* 17 (5):321–28.

Shah, H. A., L. F. Paszat, R. Saskin, T. A. Stukel, and L. Rabeneck. 2007. Factors associated with incomplete colonoscopy: A population-based study. *Gastroenterology* 132 (7):2297–2303.

Shah, R., S. Sabanathan, J. Richardson, A. J. Mearns, and C. Goulden. 1996. Results of surgical treatment of stage I and II lung cancer. *Journal of Cardiovascular Surgery* 37 (2):169–72.

Sharoni, Y., M. Danilenko, and J. Levy. 2000. Molecular mechanisms for the anticancer activity of the carotenoid lycopene. *Drug Development Research* 50 (3–4):448–56.

Shimizu, J., U. Wada-Funada, H. Mano, Y. Matahira, M. Kawaguchi, and M. Wada. 2005. Proportion of murine cytotoxic T cells is increased by high molecular-weight fucoidan extracted from Okinawa mozuku (*Cladosiphon okamuranus*). *Journal of Health Sciences* 51:394–97.

Shishodia, S., H. M. Amin, R. Lai, and B. B. Aggarwal. 2005. Curcumin (diferuloylmethane) inhibits constitutive NF-kappaB activation, induces G1/S arrest, suppresses proliferation, and induces apoptosis in mantle cell lymphoma. *Biochemical Pharmacology* 70 (5):700–13.

Shoba, G., D. Joy, T. Joseph, M. Majeed, R. Rajendran, and P. S. Srinivas. 1998. Influence of piperine on the pharmacokinetics of curcumin in animals and human volunteers. *Planta Medica* 64 (4):353–6.

Sies, H., and W. Stahl. 1998. Lycopene: Antioxidant and biological effects and its bioavailability in the human. *Proceedings of the Society for Experimental Biology and Medicine* 218 (2):121–24.

Silveira, E. M., M. F. Rodrigues, M. S. Krause, D. R. Vianna, B. S. Almeida, J. S. Rossato, L. P. Oliveira Jr., R. Curi, and P. de Bittencourt Jr. 2007. Acute exercise stimulates macrophage function: Possible role of NF-kappaB pathways. *Cell Biochemistry and Function* 25 (1):63–73.

Simon, S. 2006. Le terrain et les vaccins. *Biocontact* 163:28.

Simone, C. B., N. L. Simone, and C. B. Simone II. 1997. Oncology care augmented with nutritional and lifestyle modification. *Journal of Orthomolecular Medicine* 12 (4):197–206.

Simone II, C. B., N. L. Simone, V. Simone, and C. B. Simone. 2007. Antioxidants and other nutrients do not interfere with chemotherapy or radiation therapy and can increase kill and increase survival, part 1. *Alternative Therapies in Health and Medicine* 13 (1–2):22–28, 40–47.

Simonsen, N. R., N. J. Fernandez-Crehuet Navajas, J. M. Martin-Moreno, J. J. Strain, J. K. Huttunen, B. C. Martin, M. Thamm, A. F. Kardinaal, P. van't Veer, F. J. Kok, and L. Kohlmeier. 1998. Tissue stores of individual monounsaturated fatty acids and breast cancer: The EURAMIC study—European Community Multicenter Study on Antioxidants, Myocardial Infarction, and Breast Cancer. *American Journal of Clinical Nutrition* 68 (1):134–41.

Simonton, O. C., S. Matthews-Simonton, and J. L. Creighton. 1992. *Getting Well Again.* New York: Bantam.

Simonton, O. C., S. Matthews-Simonton, and T. F. Sparks. 1980. Psychological intervention in the treatment of cancer. *Psychosomatics* 21 (3):226–27, 231–33.

Simopoulos, A. P. 1999. Essential fatty acids in health and chronic disease. *American Journal of Clinical Nutrition* 70 (Suppl. 3):560S–69S.

———. 2002. Omega-3 fatty acids in inflammation and autoimmune diseases. *Journal of the American College of Nutrition* 21(6):495–505.

———. 2008. The importance of the omega-6/omega-3 fatty acid ratio in cardiovascular disease and other chronic diseases. *Experimental Biology and Medicine* 233 (6):674–88.

Smith, H. J., E. A. Gaffan, and P. J. Rogers. 2004. Methylxanthines are the psycho-pharmacologically active constituents of chocolate. *Psychopharmacology* 176 (3–4):412–19.

Smith, J. E., N. J. Rowan, and R. Sullivan. 2002. *Medicinal mushrooms: Their therapeutic properties and current medical usage with special emphasis on cancer treatments.* London: Cancer Research UK. http://sci.cancer-researchuk.org/labs/med_mush/med_mush.html.

Smith, J. S., F. Ameri, and P. Gadgil. 2008. Effect of marinades on the formation of heterocyclic amines in grilled beef steaks. *Journal of Food Science* 73 (6):T100–05.

Snowdon, D. A., R. L. Phillips, and W. Choi. 1984. Diet, obesity, and risk of fatal prostate cancer. *American Journal of Epidemiology* 120 (2):244–50.

Sogyal Rinpoche. 1992. *The Tibetan Book of Living and Dying.* San Francisco: Harper.

Solomon, S. D., E. T. Gerrity, and A. M. Muff. 1992. Efficacy of treatments for posttraumatic stress disorder: An empirical review. *Journal of the American Medical Association* 268 (5):633–38.

Sood, A., and T. J. Moynihan. 2005. Cancer-related fatigue: An update. *Current Oncology Reports* 7 (4):277–82.

Sørensen, T. I., G. G. Nielsen, P. K. Andersen, and T. W. Teasdale. 1988. Genetic and environmental influences on premature death in adult adoptees. *New England Journal of Medicine* 318 (12):727–32.

Speca, M., L. E. Carlson, E. Goodey, and M. Angen. 2000. A randomized, wait-list controlled clinical trial: The effect of a mindfulness, meditation-based stress reduction program on mood and symptoms of stress in cancer outpatients. *Psychosomatic Medicine* 62 (5):613–22.

Steliarova-Foucher, E., C. Stiller P. Kaatsch, F. Berrino, J. W. Coebergh, B. Lacour, and M. Perkin. 2004. Geographical patterns and time trends of cancer incidence and survival among children and adolescents in Europe since the 1970s (the ACCIS project): An epidemiological study. *Lancet* 364 (9451):2097–105.

Steptoe, A., K. O'Donnell, E. Badrick, M. Kumari, and M. Marmot. 2008. Neuroendocrine and inflammatory factors associated with positive affect in healthy men and women: The Whitehall II study. *American Journal of Epidemiology* 167 (1):96–102.

Sternberg, E. M., G. P. Chrousos, R. L. Wilder, and P. W. Gold. 1992. The stress response and the regulation of inflammatory disease. *Annals of Internal Medicine* 117 (10):854–66.

Stewart, B. W., and P. Kleihues, eds. 2003. *World Cancer Report 2003.* Lyon, France: IARC Press.

Stoneham, M., M. Goldacre, V. Seagroatt, and L. Gill. 2000. Olive oil, diet, and colorectal cancer: An ecological study and a hypothesis. *Journal of Epidemiology and Community Health* 54 (10):756–60.

Strauman, T. J., A. M. Lemieux, and C. L. Coe. 1993. Self-discrepancy and natural killer cell activity: Immunological consequences of negative self-evaluation. *Journal of Personality and Social Psychology* 64 (6):1042–52.

Streitberger, K., J. Ezzo, and A. Schneider. 2006. Acupuncture for nausea and vomiting: An update of clinical and experimental studies. *Autonomic Neuroscience: Basic and Clinical* 129 (1–2):107–17.

Su, L. J., and L. Arab. 2001. Nutritional status of folate and colon cancer risk: Evidence from NHANES I epidemiological follow-up study. *Annals of Epidemiology* 11 (1):65–72.

Sun, Y., Y. Chang, and G. Yu. 1981. Effect of fu-zheng therapy in the management of malignant diseases. *Chinese Medical Journal* 61 (97):97–101.

Sun, Y., T. J. Gan, J. W. Dubose, and A. S. Habib. 2008. Acupuncture and related techniques for postoperative pain: A systematic review of randomized controlled trials. *British Journal of Anaesthesia* 101 (2):151–60.

Tanaka, Y., S. Inoue, and S. C. Skoryna. 1970. Studies on inhibition of intestinal absorption of radioactive strontium IX: Relationship between biological activity and electron microscopic appearance of alginic acid components. *Canadian Medical Association Journal* 103 (5):484–86.

Tassman, G. C., J. N. Zafran, and G. M. Zayon. 1964. Evaluation of a plant proteolytic enzyme for the control of inflammation and pain. *Journal of Dental Medicine* 19:73–77.

Taylor, P. A. 2007. Eat organic and live longer. *Health Freedom News* 25 (4):5.

Tchekmedyian, N., J. Kallich, A. McDermott, S. Fayers, and M. Erder. 2003. The relationship between psychological stress and cancer-related fatigue. *Cancer* 98 (1):198–203.

Tei, C., Y. Horikiri, J. C. Park, J. W. Jeong, K. S. Chang, Y. Toyama, and N. Tanaka. 1995. Acute hemodynamic improvement by thermal vasodilatation in congestive heart failure. *Circulation* 91 (10):2582–90.

Tei, C., and N. Tanaka. 1996. Thermal vasodilatation as a treatment of congestive heart failure: A novel approach. *Journal of Cardiology* 27 (1):29–30.

Temoshok, L. 1987. Personality, coping style, emotion, and cancer: Towards an integrative model. *Cancer Surveys* 6 (3):545–67.

Thaker, P. H., L. Y. Han, A. A. Kamat, J. M. Arevalo, R. Takahashi, C. Lu, N. B. Jennings, G. Armaiz-Pena, J. A. Bankson, M. Ravoori, W. M. Merritt, Y. G. Lin, L. S. Mangala, T. J. Kim, R. L. Coleman, C. N. Landen, Y. Li, E. Felix, A. M. Sanguino, R. A. Newman, M. Lloyd, D. M. Gershenson, V. Kundra, G. Lopez-Berestein, S. K. Lutgendorf, S. W. Cole, and A. K. Sood. 2006. Chronic stress promotes tumor growth and angiogenesis in a mouse model of ovarian carcinoma. *Nature Medicine* 12 (8):939–44.

Thompson, L. U., J. M. Chen, T. Li, K. Strasser-Weippl, and P. E. Goss. 2005. Dietary flaxseed alters tumor biological markers in postmenopausal breast cancer. *Clinical Cancer Research* 11 (10):3828–35.

Thomson, M., and M. Ali. 2003. Garlic (*Allium sativum*): A review of its potential use as an anticancer agent. *Current Cancer Drug Targets* 3 (1):67–81.

Thomson, M., K. K. Al-Qattan, T. Bordia, and M. Ali. 2006. Including garlic in the diet may help lower blood glucose, cholesterol, and triglycerides. *Journal of Nutrition* 136 (Suppl. 3):800S–02.

Thune, I., and A. S. Furberg. 2001. Physical activity and cancer risk: Dose response and cancer, all sites and site-specific. *Medicine and Science in Sports and Exercise* 33 (Suppl. 6):S530–50.

Toyokuni, S., K. Okamoto, J. Yodoi, and H. Hiai. 1995. Persistent oxidative stress in cancer. *FEBS Letters* 358 (1):1–3.

Ulvik, A., S. E. Vollset, G. Hoff, and P. M. Ueland. 2008. Coffee consumption and circulating B-vitamins in healthy middle-aged men and women. *Clinical Chemistry* 54 (9):1489–96.

U.S. Department of Agriculture (USDA) Human Nutrition Information Service. Exler J., J. L. Wehrauch. 1988. Provisional table on the content of omega-3 fatty acids and other fat components in selected foods. U.S.D.A. Human Nutrition Information Service, HNS/PT-103.

U.S. Environmental Protection Agency. 1993. Fact sheet: Respiratory health effects of passive smoking. Office of Research and Development, and Office of Air and Radiation. EPA document no. 43-F-93-003. www.epa.gov/smokefree/pubs/etsfs.html (accessed May 15, 2009).

———. 1998. Great lakes binational toxics strategy: Stakeholder forum 1998—Implementing the Binational Toxics Strategy Polychlorinated Biphenyls (PCBs) Workgroup. www.epa.gov/glnpo/bnsdocs/pcbsrce/pcbsrce.html.

U.S. Food and Drug Administration. 2006. Mercury levels in commercial fish and shellfish. www.cfsan.fda.gov/~frf/sea-mehg.html (accessed May 14, 2009).

Van Baalen, D., M. J. de Vries, and M. T. Gondrie. 1987. Psychosocial correlates of "spontaneous" regression in cancer. Monograph, Department of General Pathology, Medical Faculty, Erasmus University, Rotterdam, the Netherlands.

Van Lommel, P., R. van Wees, V. Meyers, and I. Elfferich. 2001. Near-death experience in survivors of cardiac arrest: A prospective study in the Netherlands. *Lancet* 358 (9298):2039–45.

Van Poppel, G., D. T. Verhoeven, H. Verhagen, and R. A. Goldbohm. 1999. Brassica vegetables and cancer prevention: Epidemiology and mechanisms. *Advances in Experimental Medicine and Biology* 471:159–68.

Veterans Health Administration and Department of Defense. 2004. *VA/DoD clinical practice guideline for the management of post-traumatic stress. Version 1.* Washington, DC: Veterans Health Administration and Department of Defense.

Vickers, A. J., F. J. Bianco, A. M. Serio, J. A. Eastham, D. Schrag, E. A. Klein, A. M. Reuther, M. W. Kattan, J. E. Pontes, P. T. Scardino. 2007. The surgical learning curve for prostate cancer control after radical prostatectomy. *Journal of the National Cancer Institute* 99 (15):1171–77.

Vinzenz, K. 1991. Double blind trial on using proteolytic enzymes in dental surgery. [In German.] *Die Quintessenz* 7:1053.

Visintainer, M. A., J. R. Volpicelli, and M. E. Seligman. 1982. Tumor rejection in rats after inescapable or escapable shock. *Science* 216 (4544):437–39.

Wadleigh, R. G., R. S. Redman, M. L. Graham, S. H. Krasnow, A. Anderson, and M. H. Cohen. 1992. Vitamin E in the treatment of chemotherapy-induced mucositis. *American Journal of Medicine* 92 (5):481–84.

Walaszek, Z., M. Hanausek, J. Szemraj, and A. K. Adams. 1998. D-Glucaric acid as a prospective tumor marker. In *Tumor marker protocols*, ed. M. Hanausek, Z. Walaszek. Totowa, NJ: Humana Press, 487–95.

Walker, E. M., A. I. Rodriguez, B. Kohn, J. Pegg, R. M. Bell, and R. A. Levine. 2008. Acupuncture for the treatment of vasomotor symptoms in breast cancer patients receiving hormone suppression treatment. *International Journal of Radiation Oncology, Biology, and Physics* 72 (Suppl. 1):S103.

Wallace, J. M. 2002. Nutritional and botanical modulation of the inflammatory cascade—eicosanoids, cyclooxygenases, and lipoxygenases—as an adjunct in cancer therapy. *Integrative Cancer Therapies* 1 (1):7–37.

Wang, C. C., ed. 2000. *Clinical Radiation Oncology: Indications, Techniques, and Results.* 2nd ed. New York: Wiley-Liss.

Warburg, O. 1966. The prime cause and prevention of cancer. English ed. Presentation at meeting of Nobel Laureates, Landau, Germany, June 30. Available at www.stopcancer.com/ottolecture3.htm (accessed May 11, 2009).

Warren, R. 2002. *The Purpose Driven Life.* Grand Rapids, MI: Zondervan.

Wassef, F. 1998. Astragalus: Spanning Eastern and Western medicine. *American Journal of Natural Medicine* 5 (5):26.

Webb, A. R., L. Kline, and M. F. Holick. 1988. Influence of season and latitude on the cutaneous synthesis of vitamin D3: Exposure to winter sunlight in Boston and Edmonton will not promote vitamin D3 synthesis in human skin. *Journal of Clinical Endocrinology and Metabolism* 67 (2):373–78.

Wei, H., R. Sun, W. Xiao, J. Feng, C. Zhen, X. Xu, and Z. Tian. 2003. Traditional Chinese medicine Astragalus reverses predominance of Th2 cytokines and their up-stream transcript factors in lung cancer patients. *Oncology Reports* 10:1507–12.

Weiderpass, E., G. Gridley, I. Persson, O. Nyrén, A. Ekbom, and H. O. Adami. 1997. Risk of endometrial and breast cancer in patients with diabetes mellitus. *International Journal of Cancer* 71 (3):360–63.

Weill, P., B. Schmitt, G. Chesneau, N. Daniel, F. Safraou, and P. Legrand. 2002. Effects of introducing linseed in livestock diet on blood fatty acid composition of consumers of animal products. *Annals of Nutrition and Metabolism* 46 (5):182–91.

Whiteside, T. L., and R. B. Herberman. 1990. Characteristics of natural killer cells and lymphocyte-activated killer cells. *Immunology and Allergy Clinics of North America* 10:663–704.

Whyche, S. 2007. Modafinil relieves cognitive chemotherapy side effects. *Psychiatric News* 42(15):31.

Witek-Janusek, L., K. Albuquerque, K. R. Chroniak, C. Chroniak, R. Durazo-Arvizu, and H. L. Mathews. 2008. Effect of mindfulness-based stress reduction on immune function, quality of life, and coping in women newly diagnosed with early stage breast cancer. *Brain, Behavior, and Immunity* 22 (6):969–81.

Wollowski, I., G. Rechkemmer, and B. L. Pool-Zobel. 2001. Protective role of probiotics and prebiotics in colon cancer. *American Journal of Clinical Nutrition* 73 (2 Suppl.):451S–55S.

Won, J. S. 2002. The hematoimmunologic effect of AHCC for Korean patients with various cancers. *Biotherapy* 16 (6):560–64.

Wood, L. A. 1985. Possible prevention of adriamycin-induced alopecia by tocopherol. *New England Journal of Medicine* 312 (16):1060.

Woolery, A., H. Myers, B. Sternlieb, and L. Zeltzer. 2004. A yoga intervention for young adults with elevated symptoms of depression. *Alternative Therapies in Health and Medicine* 10 (2):60–63.

World Cancer Research Fund. 2007. WCRF/AICR Expert Report: *Food, nutrition, physical activity and the prevention of cancer: A global perspective.* Companion report: *Policy and Action for Cancer Prevention.* http://www.dietandcancerreport.org/

World Cancer Research Fund. 2009. WCRF/AICR Expert Report: *Food, nutrition, physical activity and the prevention of cancer: A global perspective.* http://dietandcancerreport.org/

Wyshak, G., and R. E. Frisch. 1994. Carbonated beverages, dietary calcium, the dietary calcium/phosphorus ratio, and bone fractures in girls and boys. *Journal of Adolescent Health* 15 (3):210–15.

Xie, X., W. Xia, Z. Li, H.-P. Kuo, Y. Liu, Z. Li, Q. Ding, S. Zhang, B. Spohn, Y. Yang, Y. Wei, J.-Y. Lang, D. B. Evans, P. J. Chiao, J. L. Abbruzzese, and M.-C. Hung. 2007. Targeted expression of BikDD eradicates pancreatic tumors in noninvasive imaging models. *Cancer Cell* 12 (1):52–65.

Yatani, R., T. Shiraishi, K. Nakakuki, I. Kusano, H. Takanari, T. Hayashi, and G. N. Stemmermann. 1988. Trends in frequency of latent prostate carcinoma in Japan from 1965–1979 to 1982–1986. *Journal of the National Cancer Institute* 80 (9):683–87.

Yun, T. K., S. Y. Choi, and H. Y. Yun. 2001. Epidemiological study on cancer prevention by ginseng: Are all kinds of cancers preventable by ginseng? *Journal of Korean Medical Science* 16 Suppl.:S19–27.

Zauber, A. G., M. J. O'Brien, and S. J. Winawer. 2002. On finding flat adenomas: Is the search worth the gain? *Gastroenterology* 122 (3):839–40.

Zhdanova, I. V., and R. J. Wurtman. 1997. The pineal hormone: Melatonin. In *Endocrinology: Basic and Clinical Principles*, ed. P. M. Conn and S. Melmed, 279–90. Totowa, NJ: Humana Press.

Zohar, J., R. Sonnino, A. Juven-Wetzler, and H. Cohen. 2009. Can posttraumatic stress disorder be prevented? *CNS spectrums* 14 (Suppl. 1):44–51.

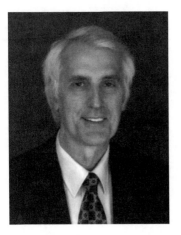

**Dan Kenner, Ph.D., L.Ac.,** is a consultant in alternative health care with more than thirty years of clinical experience in Chinese, Japanese, and naturopathic medicine. He has consulted with cancer patients for more than twenty-five years on immune restoration and finding resources for longevity and well-being. Kenner trained and completed internships in Japan and is licensed to practice oriental medicine both in Japan and the United States. He is on the board of governors of the National Health Federation and consults with clinics and companies on various aspects of alternative health care. Look online for research updates and information on longevity tools at www.dankennerresearch.com.

Foreword writer **EnRico Melson, MD,** is executive director of Global Integrative Medicine Network and chairman, CEO, and health officer of AHA! Ventures, Inc. He has undergone postdoctoral training at Memorial Sloan-Kettering Cancer Center of Cornell University, consults in the health, business, spiritual, and educational communities and speaks internationally on health issues.

# Index

vision quest, 127

visualization, 121, 126

vitamins: folate, 73; synthetic vs. natural, 70-71; vitamin A, 58; vitamin B12, 136; vitamin C, 40, 68-69; vitamin D, 75, 80-81; vitamin E, 55, 69-70, 134, 136, 138. *See also* supplements

vomiting. *See* nausea and vomiting

## W

"War on Cancer," 4

Warburg, Otto, 8, 44, 90

Warren, Rick, 124

water filtration, 36, 86

weakness and fatigue, 135

Web resources, 141-142

weight issues, 46, 80, 134-135

white blood cells, 10

white flour, 44-45

wine, 33, 62

writing, 110

## X

xenoestrogens, 60

X-rays, 82-83

## Y

yoga, 93, 126

*You Can Conquer Cancer: Prevention and Management* (Gawler), 122

## Z

zinc, 40, 74

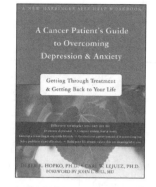
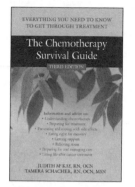
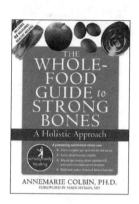
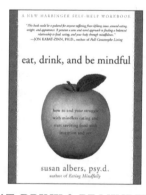
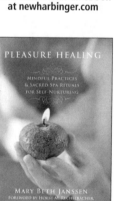
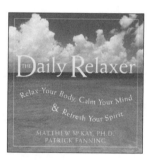
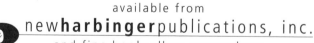